Motherhood and Postnatal Depression

Carolyn Westall • Pranee Liamputtong

Motherhood and Postnatal Depression

Narratives of Women and Their Partners

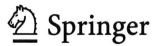 Springer

Carolyn Westall
Peace of Mind Parenting Support
P.O. Box 3126
Eltham, Victoria
Australia
westallcarolyn@yahoo.com.au

Pranee Liamputtong
School of Public Health
La Trobe University
Bundoora Victoria
Melbourne, Australia
pranee@latrobe.edu.au

ISBN 978-94-007-1693-3   e-ISBN 978-94-007-1694-0
DOI 10.1007/978-94-007-1694-0
Springer Dordrecht Heidelberg London New York

Library of Congress Control Number: 2011934263

Printed on acid-free paper

Springer is part of Springer Science+Business Media (www.springer.com)

This book is dedicated to five special people. Sue, Carolyn's sister, tragically died in the Black Saturday bushfires in Victoria, Australia, along with Sue's partner, Bob O'Sullivan, Sue's son, Jon, and two friends. The bushfires were the worst in Australia's history, and have had a devastating impact on our community.

Preface

Becoming a mother is not just a physical event and emotional milestone; it is a time of emotional adjustment and changes the family dynamics. The adjustment to motherhood is powerfully shaped by women's social interactions with others and support is crucial to this adjustment. Although motherhood brings joy to most mothers, some women may experience difficulties associated with motherhood. One of the reasons for this is their experience of postnatal depression (PND) (Wilkinson and Mulcahy 2010).

Postnatal depression (PND) affects 10–15% of women in Western society (O'Hara and Swain 1996). In Australia, PND affects 14% of women (Buist et al. 2006), and antenatal depression affects 10% of pregnant women (Beyond Blue 2010). Feminist sociologists, however, argue that PND is socially constructed and view PND as a normal response to motherhood (Berggren-Clive 1998; Brown et al. 1994; Kitzinger 1992; Mauthner 1993, 1995, 1999, 2002; Nicolson 1986, 1990; WHO 2000).

The central argument throughout this book is the importance of support before and after the birth for women's emotional well-being. This book includes women's journeys through pregnancy, childbirth, motherhood, postnatal depression, and recovery. To date, literature has focused on women's lived experiences of postnatal depression rather than their personal journeys through pregnancy, childbirth, and early motherhood. Additionally, the adjustment to fatherhood has received less attention (Condon et al. 2004). For example, little is known about the impact of postnatal depression on the partner, what support partners offer when women are diagnosed with postnatal depression, or the emotional well-being of partners after the birth.

This book intends to fill the gap in knowledge of cultural and social issues relating to pregnancy, childbirth, and motherhood for women who were diagnosed with, and had resolved, postnatal depression. Data presented in this proposed book derive from an empirical research which involved in-depth interviews and drawings from 33 women who resolved PND, and 18 partners in Melbourne, Australia. The partners' experiences added richness to the women's stories and drawings.

Carolyn's interest in PND is both personal and professional. She experienced PND after her second child. Over a period of months she feared she would hurt herself or her children. It was this fear that prompted her to seek help, initially from her general practitioner, then later from a psychologist. After 6 months of antidepressant medication and individual counselling, she is now happy to say that her experience of PND is now in the past.

Carolyn also has professional experience with PND working as a maternal and child health nurse. As a maternal and child health nurse she was in contact with large numbers of women who openly told her about their attempts to smother, throw, shake, or strangle their babies. Some women also tried to kill themselves to escape the misery that represented motherhood for them. Many of these women were in desperate need of help, and even when they were receiving treatment, they continued to be depressed. Carolyn has also been facilitating PND support groups since 2001 and has seen the benefit of connecting women to share their honest feelings about motherhood.

This book is relevant to families contemplating pregnancy, or families with children, and also health professionals caring for women in the antenatal and postnatal period, such as midwives, obstetricians, general practitioners, maternal and child health nurses, pediatricians, counsellors, psychologists, child birth educators, and mental health nurses. What we present in this book could be used to inform and develop programs to identify women who are particularly vulnerable to experiencing PND, or to improve the treatment of the illness to assist other families in their recovery.

At present, most books about parenthood were written about a decade ago, focus on women's lived experience of postnatal depression, not women's individual journeys prior to diagnosis. Women's drawings of postnatal depression and resolution could not be found in the literature, and little is known about the partner's experience of postnatal depression in women. In this book, we offer readers with our empirical data gathered from the women and their partners. We offer much more than the previous books and these include the women's stories, their partners, and an innovative research method in the health and social sciences (drawing method).

In bringing this book to life, we are grateful to several people. First we would like to thank the participants who spoke so honestly about their difficult experiences and the sensitive topic of PND. Second, we would like to acknowledge the support from Dr. Phil Maude, Associate Professor Marilys Guillemin, Professor Anne Buist at the University of Melbourne, and the University of Melbourne for the scholarship they provided for Carolyn's PhD. Third, we would like to thank Esther Otten, senior acquisition editor of Springer Publishing company for her on-going support with publishing this book. Fourth, Carolyn would like to thank her husband, Kyle, and children, her mother, Vicky, and other friends and family for their support. Pranee would like to thank Carolyn who invited her to take part in bringing this book to life. She also wishes to thank her two daughters for being part of her experience of motherhood. Pranee suffered a mild form of PND in the first few months of her first baby. Through intense support of her mother, Yindee Liamputtong, who travelled from Thailand to help her take care of the baby and other household chores, Pranee recovered quickly. Pranee wishes to express her utmost thanks to her mother for her ongoing support.

Some of the material presented in Chaps. 6 and 8 also appears in Guillemin and Westall (2007).

Melbourne   Carolyn Westall and Pranee Liamputtong

References

Berggren-Clive, K. (1998). Out of the darkness and into the light: Women's experiences with depression of childbirth. *Canadian Journal of Community Mental Health, 17*, 103–120.

Beyond Blue. (2010). What is postnatal depression? http://www.beyondblue.org.au/index. aspx?link_id=94. Accessed 28 May 2010.

Brown, S., Lumley, J., Small, R., & Astbury, J. (1994). *Missing voices. The experience of motherhood.* Australia: Oxford University Press.

Guillemin, M., & Westall, C. (2007). Gaining insight into women's knowing of postnatal depression using drawings. In P. Liamputtong, & J. Rumbold (Eds.), *Knowing differently: An introduction to experiential and arts-based research methods.* New York: Nova Science Publishers.

Kitzinger, S. (1992). *Ourselves as mothers. The universal experience of motherhood.* London: Doubleday.

Mauthner, N. S. (1993). Towards a feminist understanding of 'postnatal depression'. *Feminism and Psychology, 3*(3), 350–355.

Mauthner, N. S. (1995). Postnatal depression: The significance of social contacts between mothers. *Women's Studies International Forum, 18*, 311–323.

Mauthner, N. S. (1999). Feeling low and feeling really bad about feeling low: Women's experiences of motherhood and postpartum depression. *Canadian Psychology, 40*(2), 143–161.

Mauthner, N. S. (2002). *The darkest days of my life. Stories of postpartum depression.* Cambridge: Harvard University Press.

Nicolson, P. (1986). Developing a feminist approach to depression following childbirth. In S. Wilkinson (Ed.), *Feminist social psychology: Developing theory and practice.* Philadelphia: Open University Press.

Nicolson, P. (1990). Understanding postnatal depression: A mother-centred approach. *Journal of Advanced Nursing, 15*, 689–695.

O'Hara, M. W., & Swain, A. M. (1996). Rates and risk of postpartum depression – A meta-analysis. *International Review of Psychiatry, 8*, 37–54.

WHO. (2000). *Women's mental health. An evidenced based review.* Geneva: WHO.

Wilkinson, R. B., & Mulcahy, R. (2010). Attachment and interpersonal relationships in postnatal depression. *Journal of Reproductive and Infant Psychology, 28*(3), 252–265.

About the Authors

Carolyn Westall is a parenting consultant for Peace of Mind Parenting Support which provides assistance to families who are struggling or need additional support with parenting. She is a registered nurse, midwife, and maternal and child health nurse who has facilitated postnatal support groups since 2001. For her Ph.D. Carolyn interviewed 33 women who resolved postnatal depression, and 18 partners; the research on which this book is based. She has two children, Erin and Conor.

Carolyn is passionate about trying to prevent postnatal depression and to help people with their emotional recovery following major disasters. To follow this passion, Carolyn has set up a charity, the Sue Evans Fund for Families, in memory of her sister (see dedication page at the front of the book). For more information go to www.sueevansfund.com.au

Carolyn has published one chapter in a book: Gaining insight into women's knowing of postnatal depression using drawings (with Marilys Guillemin). In P. Liamputtong and J. Rumbold (Eds.). *Knowing Differently: An Introduction to Experiential and Arts-Based Research Methods* (Nova Science Publishers, 2007). She has also published one journal article about postnatal depression: *Childbirth and postnatal depression, Birth Matters* (2002).

Pranee Liamputtong holds a Personal Chair in Public Health at the School of Public Health, La Trobe University, Melbourne, Australia. Pranee has previously taught in the School of Sociology and Anthropology and worked as a public health research fellow at the Centre for the Study of Mothers' and Children's Health (now Mothers and Child Health Research), La Trobe University. Pranee's particular interests include issues related to cultural and social influences on childbearing, childrearing, and women's reproductive and sexual health. Pranee has two daughters, Zoe and Emma.

Pranee has published several books and a large number of papers in these areas. These include: *Maternity and Reproductive Health in Asian Societies* (with Lenore Manderson, Harwood Academic Press, 1996); *Asian Mothers, Western Birth* (Ausmed Publications, 1999); *Living in a New Country: Understanding Migrants' Health* (Ausmed Publications, 1999); *Hmong Women and Reproduction* (Bergin and

Garvey 2000); *Coming of Age in South and Southeast Asia: Youth, Courtship and Sexuality* (with Lenore Manderson, Curzon Press, 2002); *Health, Social Change and Communities* (with Heather Gardner, Oxford University Press, 2003). Her more recent books include *Reproduction, Childbearing and Motherhood: A Cross-Cultural Perspective* (Nova Science Publishers, 2007); *Childrearing and Infant Care Issues: A Cross-Cultural Perspective* (Nova Science Publishers, 2007); *The Journey of Becoming a Mother amongst Thai Women in Northern Thailand* (Lexington Books, 2007); *Population, Community, and Health Promotion* (with Sansnee Jirojwong, Oxford University Press, 2008); *Infant Feeding Practices: A Cross-Cultural Perspective* (Springer, New York, 2010); and *Health, Illness and Well-Being: Perspectives and Social Determinants* (with Rebecca Fanany and Glenda Verrinder, Oxford University Press, Melbourne, in press). She is in the process of editing two books in HIV/AIDS from a cross-cultural perspective for Springer.

Pranee has published several research method books. Her first research method book is titled *Qualitative Research Methods: A Health Focus* (with Douglas Ezzy, Oxford University Press, 1999, reprinted in 2000, 2001, 2003, 2004); the second edition of this book is titled *Qualitative Research Methods* (2005, reprinted in 2006, 2007, 2008); and the third edition is authored solely by herself (*Qualitative Research Methods, 3rd edition*, 2009). Pranee has also published a book on doing qualitative research online: *Health Research in Cyberspace: Methodological, Practical and Personal Issues* (Nova Science Publishers, 2006). Her new books include *Researching the Vulnerable: A Guide to Sensitive Research Methods* (Sage, London, 2007); *Undertaking Sensitive Research: Managing Boundaries, Emotions and Risk* (with Virginia Dickson-Swift and Erica James, Cambridge University Press, 2008); *Knowing Differently: Arts-Based and Collaborative Research Methods* (with Jean Rumbold, Nova Science Publishers, 2008); *Doing Cross-Cultural Research: Ethical and Methodological Issues* (Springer, 2008); *Performing Qualitative Cross-Cultural Research* (Cambridge University Press, 2010), and *Research Methods in Health: Foundations for Evidence-Based Practice* (Oxford University Press, 2010). Her most recent book is *Focus Group Methodology: Principle and Practice* (Sage, 2011).

Contents

Chapter 1
Introduction: From Pregnancy to Resolution from Postnatal Depression

The bad thoughts came back again. I was imagining drowning the kids in the pool and then going up to the high-rise and just jumping off. I've never actually told anyone that before. That's when I said to Nathan [husband], "You need to get me some help and I don't care who it is [or] what they do- whether it's acupuncture or alternative, something. I don't want to go back on medication". He was good, he went out and came home from work that night and said, "I've got the number of a guy [complementary therapist]. I've booked you in, and I'll take you on Saturday" (Mary).

Mary experienced postnatal depression (PND) three times – after each of her children's births. She referred to her first two episodes as "mild" which required no treatment. Following the birth of Mary's third baby, she knew she had PND. This episode of PND was the most severe of the three episodes, and lasted for 3 years. Antidepressant medication alone was unable to lift her depression. Mary, like many other women in our research, explained their PND as a result of their circumstances, rather than hormonal changes. This quote by Mary echoes the sentiments of most women participants as it highlights two important points. Firstly, women with PND were often in crisis when they sought help. Secondly, partners played a crucial role in supporting women by identifying symptoms and assisting women to treatment.

1.1 Motherhood and Postnatal Depression

Motherhood is a monumental achievement. Maternal role attainment was first described by Rubin (1967a, b) as a process that begins in pregnancy, and ends with the formation of a maternal identity 1 year after the birth. Mercer (1985: 198) defines maternal role attainment as 'a process in which the mother achieves competence in the role and integrates the mothering behaviours into her established role set, so that she is comfortable with her identity as a mother'. The 'normal' adjustment to motherhood has been explored extensively in the literature, especially for first-time mothers (Barclay et al. 1997; Liamputtong 2006, 2007; Mercer 1986, 2004;

C. Westall and P. Liamputtong, *Motherhood and Postnatal Depression: Narratives of Women and Their Partners*, DOI 10.1007/978-94-007-1694-0_1,
© Springer Science+Business Media B.V. 2011

Rogan et al. 1997; Rubin 1967a, b). However, questions are raised as to what constitutes the so-called 'normal' adjustment to motherhood as opposed to symptoms of PND.

Postnatal depression is caused by a combination of biological, psychological and social factors (Morrow et al. 2008). Two models have attempted to define and explain PND: the biomedical and the sociological models (WHO 2000). Whilst the medical model has been the dominant model in treating PND (Beck 2002), it has been criticised by feminist sociologists for its inflexible definition of PND (Mauthner 1993). In contrast, the social model of health places more emphasis on the psycho-social factors that contribute to depressive symptoms such as gender, poverty, social disadvantage and social class (WHO 2000).

In Australia, health care reform has had a huge impact on the emotional well-being of mothers with shorter hospital stays and limited opportunities for women to learn about motherhood and to recover from the birth. There are also shrinking community services that focus on treatment rather than prevention. McAllister (2007: 37) highlights the inadequate mental health system in Australia:

> People who experience mental illness or psychiatric disability continue to be poorly served by an entrenched and outdated system of health care that succeeds in treating acute illness, but fails to offer adequate community education and prevention, early detection or the full range of approaches that we know facilitates recovery and rehabilitation.

Thus, it is essential that health professionals and families learn as much as possible about the factors that affect women's emotional well-being in an attempt to prevent PND, and to assist women with their adjustment to motherhood.

1.2   Postnatal Depression and Its Symptoms

The symptoms of PND include sleep or appetite changes, sadness, difficulty in coping, irritability, anxiety, negative thoughts, fear of being alone, loss of memory or confusion, loss of concentration, feeling guilty, loss of self-esteem and/or thoughts of hurting the self or the baby (Post and Antenatal Depression Association 2010). The medical model's classification of PND will be explored further in Chapter 2. It is generally accepted that the onset of symptoms of PND can occur any time in the first 12 months after childbirth (Milgrom et al. 1999; National Health and Medical Research Council 2000; Wood et al. 1997).

1.3   The Impact of PND on Men and Children

There is evidence in the literature that the emotional well-being of both partners is crucial for the physical, emotional and social development of the child (Ramchandani et al. 2005). Male partners, of women with PND, also develop depression (Areias et al. 1996; Fettling 2002; Matthey et al. 2000; Meighan et al. 1999; Ramchandani et al.

2005) and PND (Bishop 1999; Smyth 2003). In Western society, men are often discouraged from showing sadness and grief and are unlikely to seek help for their depression (Cochran and Rabinowitz 2003). Undiagnosed and untreated depression in men may account for higher rates of suicide compared with women (Cochran and Rabinowitz 2003).

The impact of PND on the child is well-documented (Beck 1995, 1996; Buist 2002; Field 1998; Goodman and Gotlib 1999; Murray et al. 2003; O'Connor et al. 2002; Ramchandani et al. 2005; Sluckin 1998). Cognitive and behavioural problems in the child at a later age are well-researched. By 1 year of age, Buist and colleagues (2002) found that children of mothers with PND are at risk of attention problems and impaired cognitive and brain function; these problems may persist until school age. Hammen and Brennan (2003), in their study of 816 children, concluded that children of depressed mothers are 20% more likely to have depression themselves (versus 10% of children of non-depressed mothers). The child's age when maternal depression started was not a significant risk factor for their development of depression (Hammen and Brennan 2003).

1.4 About This Book

This introduction has provided an overview of motherhood and PND from a global perspective and in an Australian context.

In Chapter 2, we explore the traditional medical model's classification of PND in relation to the screening and diagnosis of PND. We will critically discuss three screening tools used to diagnose PND: the Edinburgh Postnatal Depression Scale (EPDS), the Beck Depression Inventory and the Postpartum Depression Screening Scale. We argue that there are limitations to using screening tools to diagnose PND, particularly if screening is not followed with a clinical interview. The clinical interview is a way of identifying the psychosocial factors that influence women's emotional well-being. The historical development of PND as a category of mental illness and its evolution from the DSM, ICD-10 and the Research Diagnostic Criteria are also discussed.

In Chapter 3, we argue that a biopsychosocial approach is needed to fully understand PND. The biopsychosocial model provides a holistic approach to health care and is commonly used in psychiatry. We provide a discussion of the biomedical and sociological models as they provide distinct views about the development and treatment of PND. Literature from the disciplines of psychology, midwifery, medicine and nursing will be analysed to provide a thorough understanding of the phenomenon of PND.

Chapter 4 examines the care women received from health professionals in pregnancy and childbirth. The lack of support women received from health professionals resulted in the loss of self-esteem and sense of failure that women experienced. Also, the insufficient amount of information about PND that couples received antenatally resulted in the difficulty identifying symptoms after the birth.

Chapter 5 explores the social construction of motherhood and the difficult adjustment to motherhood for women in this study. When women became mothers, they felt they received insufficient support, particularly from health professionals, partners, their own and other mothers after the birth for their emotional well-being. The unmet expectations of support resulted in the loss of self-esteem and feelings of disappointment and depression. Also, the loss of self resulted from the multiple losses women experienced when they became mothers. Couples identified maternal sleep deprivation as the major trigger for PND as it contributed to severe fatigue, exhaustion, social isolation and the loss of control.

In Chapter 6, we examine couples' understanding of postnatal depression, and the process of screening and diagnosis. Most women disagreed with their medical diagnosis of PND, and considered that their circumstances attributed to their emotional state, instead of hormonal changes. On the other hand, men were more likely to agree with the diagnosis of their partner's PND. In addition to women's verbal accounts, their experiences of PND were also portrayed through their drawings, giving the sense that women felt trapped, alone in the dark. These accounts highlight the sense of helplessness that women experienced.

Chapter 7 explores the impact of PND on the partner. Partners felt helpless and were unsure how to support women when they developed PND as they were excluded from treatment plans. As a result, relationship difficulties were common as postnatal depression caused a wedge in the couple's relationship, and contributed to additional stress. Two partners were diagnosed with depression when women recovered, and two men with a history of depression noticed a worsening of symptoms when women recovered.

The last chapter, Chapter 8, explores couples' experiences with the treatment of PND how they resolved the symptoms. In this chapter, we argue that a biopsychosocial approach to treatment is necessary for women's emotional well-being. This chapter highlights the support women need to resolve depressive symptoms. Women's drawings of resolution identified the physical shift away from PND, but most drawings showed remnants of darkness that represented their bad days. In contrast to women's drawings of PND where they were trapped alone in the dark, women's drawings of resolution were filled with light, colour and represented hope, and included partners and children.

References

Areias, M. E., Kumar, R., Barros, H., & Figueiredo, E. (1996). Correlates of postnatal depression in mothers and fathers. *The British Journal of Psychiatry, 169*(1), 36–41.

Barclay, L. B., Everitt, L., Rogan, F., Schmied, V., & Wyllie, A. (1997). 'Becoming a Mother' – an analysis of women's experience of early motherhood. *Journal of Advanced Nursing, 25*, 719–728.

Beck, C. T. (1995). The effect of postpartum depression on maternal-infant interaction: A meta-analysis. *Nursing Research, 44*, 298–304.

Beck, C. T. (1996). Postpartum depressed mothers' experiences interacting with their children. *Nursing Research, 45*, 98–104.

Enter the content

Beck, C. T. (2002). Theoretical perspectives of postpartum depression and their treatment implications. *The American Journal of Maternal/Child Nursing, 27*(5), 282–287.

Bishop, L. (1999). *Postnatal depression families in turmoil.* Rushcutters Bay: Halstead press.

Buist, A. (2002). Mental health in pregnancy: The sleeping giant. *Australasian Psychiatry, 10*(3), 203–206.

Buist, A., Barnett, B., Milgrom, J., Pope, S., Condon, J. T., & Ellwood, D. A. (2002). To screen or not to screen- that is the question in perinatal depression. *The Medical Journal of Australia, 177*(7 October), 101–105.

Cochran, S., & Rabinowitz, F. E. (2003). Gender-Sensitive recommendations for assessment and treatment of depression in men. *Professional Psychology- Research & Practice, 34*(2), 132–140.

Fettling, L. (2002). *Postnatal depression. A practical guide for Australian families.* Melbourne: IP Communications.

Field, T. (1998). Maternal depression effects on infants and early interventions. *Preventative Medicine, 27*(27), 200–203.

Goodman, S. H., & Gotlib, I. H. (1999). Risk for psychopathology in the children of depressed mothers: A developmental model for understanding mechanisms of transmission. *Psychological Review, 106*, 458–490.

Hammen, C., & Brennan, P. A. (2003). Severity, chronicity, and timing of maternal depression and risk for adolescent offspring diagnoses in a community sample. *Archives of General Psychiatry, 60*, 253–258.

Liamputtong, P. (2006). Motherhood and "moral career": Discourses of good motherhood among Southeast Asian immigrant women in Australia. *Qualitative Sociology, 29*(1), 25–53.

Liamputtong, P. (2007). *The journey of becoming a mother amongst women in northern Thailand.* Lanham: Lexington Books.

Matthey, S., Barnett, B., Ungerer, J., & Waters, B. (2000). Paternal and maternal depressed mood during the transition to parenthood. *Journal of Affective Disorders, 60*, 75–85.

Mauthner, N. S. (1993). Towards a feminist understanding of 'Postnatal Depression'. *Feminism and Psychology, 3*(3), 350–355.

McAllister, M. (2007). New models of care in mental health. *Australian Nursing Journal, 14*(8), 37.

Meighan, M., Davis, M. W., Thomas, S., & Droppleman, P. G. (1999). Living with postpartum depression: The father's experience. *The American Journal of Maternal/Child Nursing, 24*(4), 202–208.

Mercer, R. T. (1985). The process of maternal role attainment over the first year. *Nursing Research, 34*, 198–204.

Mercer, R. T. (1986). *First-time motherhood: Experiences from teens to forties.* New York: Springer.

Mercer, R. T. (2004). Becoming a mother versus maternal role attainment. *Journal of Nursing Scholarship, 36*(3), 226–232.

Milgrom, J., Martin, P. R., & Negri, L. M. (1999). *Treating postnatal depression. A psychological approach for health care practitioners.* Chichester: Wiley.

Morrow, M., Smith, J., Lai, Y., & Jaswal, S. (2008). Shifting landscapes: Immigrant women and post partum depression. *Health Care for Women International, 29*(6), 593–617.

Murray, L., Cooper, P., & Hipwell, A. (2003). Mental health of parents caring for infants. *Archives of Women's Mental Health, 6*(2), 71–77.

National Health and Medical Research Council. (2000). Postnatal depression. A systematic review of published scientific literature to 1999. http://www.nhmrc.gov.au/publications/synopses/wh29syn.htm. Accessed 12 June 2007.

O'Connor, T. G., Heron, J., & Glover, V. (2002). Antenatal anxiety predicts child behavioural/emotional problems independently of postnatal depression. *Journal of the American Academy of Child and Adolescent Psychiatry, 41*(12), 1470–1477.

Post and Antenatal Depression Association. (2010). Postnatal depression. http://www.panda.org.au/practical-information/about-postnatal-depression/28-postnatal-depression?start=1. Accessed 28 May 2010.

Ramchandani, P., Stein, A., Evans, J., & O'Connor, T. G. (2005). Paternal depression in the postnatal period and child development: A prospective population study. *The Lancet, 365*, 2201–2205.

Rogan, F., Shmied, V., Barclay, L., Everett, L., & Wyllie, A. (1997). 'Becoming a mother'-developing a new theory of early motherhood. *Journal of Advanced Nursing, 25*, 877–885.

Rubin, R. (1967a). Attainment of the maternal role. Part 1. Processes. *Nursing Research, 16*, 237–245.

Rubin, R. (1967b). Attainment of the maternal role. Part II: Models and referents. *Nursing Research, 16*, 324–346.

Sluckin, A. (1998). Bonding failure: 'I don't know this baby, she's nothing to do with me'. *Clinical Child Psychology and Psychiatry, 3*(1), 11–24.

Smyth, J. (2003, November 9). New fathers not immune from postpartum depression. *Chicago Sun-Times*, p. 26.

WHO. (2000). *Women's mental health. An evidenced based review*. Geneva: WHO.

Wood, A. F., Thomas, S. P., Droppleman, P. G., & Meighan, M. (1997). The downward spiral of postpartum depression. *Maternal-Child Nursing Journal, 22*, 308–317.

Chapter 2
Detection of Postnatal Depression

> Depression is the common cold of psychopathology and has touched the lives of us all, yet
> it is probably the most dimly understood and most inadequately investigated of all the major
> forms of psychopathology (Seligman 1975: 76).

This quote by Martin Seligman, a well-respected psychologist, stated, in 1975, that depression was both common and poorly understood. Postnatal depression is often confused with other mood disorders or is not detected at all (Buist 1996; National Health and Medical Research Council 2000). Our aim in this chapter is to examine the medical model's classification of PND in relation to screening and diagnosis as it has been the dominant model in the management of PND (Beck 2002b). However, the biomedical model's understanding of PND only partially explains the illness.

In the first section, 'The historical development of PND as a distinct category', we explore the emergence of the biomedical model's DSM criteria, which are used to diagnose women with PND. It is important to include a historical perspective of DSM as it provides a platform for understanding the development of PND as a distinct diagnostic category of mental illness. We will discuss the benefits and limitations of using DSM-IV-TR for the diagnosis of PND. Using the DSM-IV-TR for diagnosis ignores the psychosocial stressors affecting an individual's emotional well-being, particularly if it is not followed up with a clinical interview. Other mood disorders that are commonly confused with PND will be discussed.

In the second section, 'Screening tools', we critically discuss three different screening tools used to identify women with depression – the Edinburgh Postnatal Depression Scale, the Beck Depression Inventory and the Postpartum Depression Screening Scale. The Edinburgh Postnatal Depression Scale is the most commonly used screening tool used to detect PND and, as a result, will be explored in detail. We argue that whilst screening tools are valuable for detecting depressive symptoms, there are also limitations if women are not followed up with a clinical interview to differentiate the presence of depressive symptoms from normal symptoms occurring in the postpartum period, such as sleep deprivation and fatigue.

In the third section, 'The clinical interview', we will discuss the benefit of interviewing women as an important step following the screening process. The clinical

C. Westall and P. Liamputtong, *Motherhood and Postnatal Depression: Narratives of Women and Their Partners*, DOI 10.1007/978-94-007-1694-0_2, © Springer Science+Business Media B.V. 2011

interview provides an opportunity for women to discuss the psychosocial factors that impact on their emotional well-being. Health professionals can use the clinical interview to focus on the individual's problems or symptoms and may assist them to resolve their identified issues (Sommers-Flanagan and Sommers-Flanagan 2003).

2.1 The Historical Development of PND as a Distinct Category of Mental Illness

The evolution of postnatal mood disorders can be traced back to the nineteenth century. In 1858, Louis Victor Marcé, a French psychiatrist, was the first to publish information about puerperal mental illness as distinct from other psychiatric disorders (Marcé society 2006). In the first three editions of the Diagnostic and Statistical Manual of Mental Disorders (DSM-I, DSM-II and DSM-III), the American Psychiatric Association failed to classify PND as a distinct disorder. DSM-I was originally developed by the American Psychiatric Association (1952) to improve the reliability of psychiatric diagnosis. It consisted of only 60 disorders. DSM-II was published by the American Psychiatric Association (1968) and separated psychoses (hallucinations, delusions, and distortions of thought) from neuroses (depression and anxiety). DSM-III (American Psychiatric Association 1980) and DSM-III-R (American Psychiatric Association 1987) had clear categories for separating normal from abnormal behaviour. However, the DSM-III also failed to classify PND as a distinct category. In the DSM-III, depression was classified as a 'major affective disorder' (American Psychiatric Association 2000). The major diagnostic categories of DSM-III were developed from the Research Diagnostic Criteria (RDC) (Spitzer et al. 1975). The RDC was used specifically by psychiatrists and was created because of the low reliability of psychiatric diagnostic procedures (Spitzer et al. 1978). The RDC consisted of inclusion and exclusion criteria for 25 categories and was a diagnostic tool that could enhance an evidence-based research approach (Meier 1979; Williams and Spitzer 1982).

Over the past two decades, PND has been categorised as a distinct form of mental illness. The International Classification of Diseases (ICD-10) (WHO 1992) classified PND as a 'mental and behavioural disorder associated with the puerperium'. This category was further divided into either mild or severe episodes. ICD-10 is used for clinical and epidemiological purposes to classify diseases and other health problems to provide the basis for national mortality statistics (WHO 2006). The ICD-10 is used alternatively to the DSM criteria. Similar to the ICD-10, the American Psychiatric Association (2000) identifies that symptoms of depression begin within 6 weeks of childbirth. The DSM-IV-TR differs from the ICD-10 as it classifies PND as a 'mood episode', and it is further classified as a 'major depressive episode' (American Psychiatric Association 2000). The DSM-IV-TR (American Psychiatric Association 2000) was updated from the DSM-IV (American Psychiatric Association 1994). However, the classification for PND remained unchanged between these editions.

In summary, the American Psychiatric Association (2000) classifies PND as a form of mental illness. The psychosocial model stands in stark contrast to the biomedical model as it highlights the personal and social factors that contribute to depression, such as the lack of support (Eaker 2005; Mauthner 2002; Paris and Dubus 2005; Ray and Hodnett 2006), loss of career (Oakley 1980), poverty (WHO 2000), and significant life events (Brown and Harris 1978, 2001; Brown et al. 1995; Harris 2001, 2003).

2.1.1   The DSM-IV-TR Criteria

According to the American Psychiatric Association's (2000) *The Diagnostic and Statistical Manual of Mental Disorders, Text Revision* (DSM-IV-TR), PND is a 'major depressive episode'. Importantly, the only difference between PND and major depression is that the specifier 'with postpartum onset' is used if symptoms begin within 4 weeks after childbirth. To meet the criteria for major depression, individuals must have five or more symptoms for 2 weeks or more; one of the symptoms must include either depressed mood or loss of interest or pleasure in most or all activities and must be present most of the day or nearly every day. The other symptoms include changes in appetite (increased or decreased), weight (gain or loss of 5% within a month) or sleep (insomnia or hypersomnia); restlessness or slowed movements; fatigue or decreased energy; feelings of worthlessness or excessive guilt; difficulty in thinking, concentrating or making decisions; or recurrent thoughts of death or suicide, with or without a plan to commit suicide (American Psychiatric Association 2000).

Although the DSM has been successful in providing consistency with the diagnosis of psychiatric diagnoses, it has also been criticised for its reductionist approach and its Western perspective of what constitutes mental illness (Eriksen and Kress 2005; Spitzer et al. 1983). Eriksen and Kress (2005) identify three limitations with using DSM-IV-TR for diagnosis: issues of stigmatisation and the failure to acknowledge the uniqueness of individuals, diagnostic categories narrowing a health professional's focus by encouraging him or her to observe behaviours that fit within a medical model of understanding and failure in the prediction of treatment outcomes or identification of underlying pathology.

2.2   Other Mood Disorders in the Postpartum Period

The medical model recognises three distinct categories of mood changes/disorders specific to the postpartum period – the baby blues, PND and puerperal psychosis. Table 2.1, *Mood changes/ disorders in the postpartum period*, highlights the differences between these conditions. The baby blues is the mildest mood change, requiring no treatment. In contrast, puerperal psychosis is the most severe of the three mood changes/disorders, often requiring hospitalisation. Postnatal depression lies between the baby blues and puerperal psychosis in terms of severity of symptoms.

Table 2.1 Mood changes/disorders after childbirth

Type of mood change/disorder	Onset of symptoms	Duration of symptoms	Treatment
Baby blues	Within days after birth	Up to two weeks	Support and reassurance
Postnatal depression	Within 12 months after birth	Months or years	Various treatments
Puerperal psychosis	Within 4 weeks after birth	Not known	Possible hospitalisation and medication

(Modified from American Psychiatric Association 2000; Milgrom et al. 1999; Wisner et al. 2002).

2.2.1 The Baby Blues (Maternity Blues)

The baby blues is a transient mood change characterised by irritability, anxiety, decreased concentration, insomnia, tearfulness and mild mood swings (Ryan and Kostaras 2005). The baby blues affects up to 80% of women and occurs within days of delivery (Fettling 2002; Milgrom et al. 1999). The blues generally resolves within two weeks of delivery (O'Hara et al. 1991) and requires only support and reassurance. Persistence of the blues for more than 2 weeks after the birth is abnormal, and the diagnosis of PND needs to be excluded. Women with severe baby blues are at risk for PND (Beck 1999).

2.2.2 Puerperal Psychosis

Puerperal psychosis is a less common but more serious condition than PND and affects 1 in 500 women (Cox and Holden 2003). Puerperal psychosis has a rapid onset (Ryan and Kostaras 2005). Symptoms include inability to sleep, confusion, agitation, delusions, hallucinations, severely disturbed mood and behaviour and being often out of touch with reality (National Health and Medical Research Council 2000). In this disturbed condition, often command hallucinations are present that may, for example, instruct women to kill their infants or women may have delusional beliefs that their infants are possessed (American Psychiatric Association 2000).

2.3 Screening Tools

This section will provide a discussion of the three most commonly used screening tools used to detect depressive symptoms. Importantly, these tools were specifically designed as screening and not diagnostic tools. There are only two tools specifically designed to screen women for PND – the Edinburgh Postnatal Depression Scale and the Postpartum Depression Screening Scale. The Beck Depression Inventory (BDI) (Beck et al. 1961) is used to detect depression, as distinct to PND, in the postpartum period. The Edinburgh Postnatal Depression Scale, the Beck Depression Inventory and the Postpartum Depression Screening Scale are all self-report scales where women complete the forms, instead of the health professional eliciting the answers. Self-report instruments measure different aspects of depression as they focus on specific symptoms (Clemmens et al. 2004).

The problem with using screening tools (Edinburgh Postnatal Depression Scale, Beck Depression Inventory, Postpartum Depression Screening Scale) and diagnostic tools (DSM-IV-TR) is that women's symptoms are reduced into boxes and their individual reasons for developing PND are ignored. A clinical interview would enable women to discuss their concerns or, perhaps, underlying factors affecting their emotional well-being. The importance of using a clinical interview for diagnosis will be discussed later in this chapter.

2.3.1   Edinburgh Postnatal Depression Scale (EPDS)

The Edinburgh Postnatal Depression Scale (Appendix A) was developed by Cox, Holden and Sagovsky in 1987. They perceived that screening instruments used to detect depression, such as the original BDI, had limitations when applied to postnatal women. Importantly, the EPDS was designed as a screening tool, not a diagnostic tool, used to detect PND (Cox et al. 1987; Cox and Holden 2003; Shakespeare 2001; Sharp and Lipsky 2002). The EPDS was designed to be used by community health workers to screen specifically for PND (Wickberg and Hwang 1996). To date, the EPDS is the most common screening tool used in the world to detect antenatal and postnatal depression (Austin 2003; Buist 2002).

The EPDS takes only 5 minutes to complete and has ten questions with four responses for each question and covers mood, sleep problems and most importantly self-harm. When explaining the tool, women are asked to select the answer that closely resembles their feelings over the past week. However, the DSM-IV-TR criteria require depressive symptoms to be present for a period of 2 weeks or more. This discrepancy could result in the over diagnosis of PND. The EPDS is based on the frequency of each symptom. For example, the question 'I have blamed myself unnecessarily when things went wrong' asks for one of the following responses: 'Yes, most of the time'; 'Yes, some of the time'; 'Not very often'; and 'No, never'. Each of the questions is scored 0–3, with the highest possible score being 30. The following quote by Oates (2003: 597) highlights the dilemma that health professionals face when women screen positively with the EPDS:

> The EPDS, given at a single point in time, is likely to sweep up not only those who are ill, but those who are temporarily ill, permanently unhappy, or even those who are simply having a bad day.

Despite its widespread use, the EPDS has been criticised for ignoring psychosocial factors that contribute to PND symptoms (Beck and Gable 2000), such as the lack of support, significant life events or chronic sleep deprivation. The scale also ignores women's intent to hurt their children.

2.3.1.1 Original Validation of the EPDS

The EPDS was validated with a sample of only 84 women in the United Kingdom. Seventy-two of these women had already been identified as being 'potentially depressed' by their health visitors when their babies were approximately 6 weeks of age (Cox et al. 1987). Twelve 'normal' women were added to the sample to prevent bias from the interviewer knowing the participants. However, as women were already identified as being 'potentially depressed', this sample was biased and not representative of the population. Most women in Cox et al.'s (1987) sample were interviewed in their homes at approximately 13 weeks postpartum and completed both the EPDS and Goldberg's Standardised Psychiatric Interview (SPI) (Goldberg et al. 1970). The Research Diagnostic Criteria (RDC) (Spitzer et al. 1975) was used to validate the EPDS. Using a cut-off score of 12.5, Cox et al. (1987) found the sensitivity of the EPDS to be 86%, the specificity, 78% and the positive predictive value, 73%.

2.3.1.2 Validation Studies

The EPDS has been translated into 23 different languages and has been validated in various populations (Cox and Holden 2003). However, the validity of the EPDS in these studies is affected by the sample size, sample population, recruitment strategies employed and the presentation of the EPDS to the mother (Cox and Holden 2003; Milgrom et al. 1999; Shakespeare 2001). The EPDS fails to acknowledge cultural differences in different populations (Shakespeare 2001). For example, sadness is expressed in different ways in different cultures (Pilgrim and Bentall 1999). Cox and Holden (2003: 23) advise health professionals to use a 'culturally appropriate diagnostic interview' when screening women from different ethnic backgrounds to avoid misdiagnosis.

Only one study has validated the EPDS in an Australian sample of women. Boyce et al. (1993) validated the EPDS in community and hospital samples of 98 women. Women completed three self-report scales – the EPDS, the General Health Questionnaire (GHQ) (Goldberg 1972) and the Pitt scale (Pitt 1968). This was followed by a structured clinical interview from the Diagnostic Interview Schedule (Robins et al. 1989) to provide a DSM-III-R (American Psychiatric Association 1987) diagnosis of major depression. When the EPDS was over 12, the sensitivity was 100% (true cases identified); the specificity was 96% (true non-cases identified); the positive predictive value was 69% (women who tested positive and developed PND); and the negative predictive value was 95% (women who tested negative did not develop PND) (Boyce et al. 1993). A psychologist presented the EPDS to women in their homes, and the timing of the EPDS varied from 2 to 29 weeks after birth.

We challenge the validity of Boyce et al.'s (1993) study due to the sample recruitment, sample size and timing of the administration of the EPDS. Firstly, the sample size of 98 was small for a quantitative study. Secondly, women were difficult to recruit from the general population and were recruited from community and hospital samples. The findings of the study reflected that women were not representative of the population as the prevalence of PND was only 4%, instead of 14% as reported in Australia. Boyce and colleagues (1993) concluded that the low incidence of PND could be explained by an over-representation of depressed women among those who refused to participate. Thirdly, women were eligible for the study only if their infants were less than 6 months of age, as clinically the onset of PND is within 12 months of childbirth. Furthermore, screening women 2 weeks after birth is problematic; according to Cox and Holden (2003) screening less than 6 weeks after birth may lead to difficulties in differentiating between PND, childbirth difficulties, sleeplessness and the adjustment to the infant. At this time, women also physically recover from birth and experience hormonal changes that could affect their emotional state.

In a systematic review of 13 published studies from 1980 to 2001, Austin and Lumley (2003) examined the properties of screening tools and their use in the antenatal and postnatal periods. Austin and Lumley (2003) found that the prevalence of PND ranged from 5.5% to as high as 31.5%, and 67% of pregnant women were identified as depressed. They concluded that no screening instruments met the criteria for routine application in the antenatal period.

2.3.1.3 Different Cut-off Scores

The validity of the EPDS is also affected by the cut-off score used to detect PND. Different cut-off scores are used in different countries. Cox and associates (1987) recommend using a cut-off of 12/13 for 'probable depression' and 9/10 for 'possible depression'. Several researchers advocate using a lower cut-off score (Cox et al. 1987; Shakespeare 2001; Wisner et al. 2002). Shakespeare (2001) suggests that a lower cut-off score is used in the United Kingdom to increase the sensitivity of the EPDS; however, it creates a huge burden on health services. Oates (2003) argues that using lower cut-off scores reduces the specificity of the EPDS to 30–70%. However, other researchers assert that a lower cut-off score is necessary for reliability (Wisner et al. 2002) to reduce failed detection to less than 10% (Cox et al. 1987) and to reduce the chance of false positive results (Buist et al. 2002).

Despite the cut-off scores used when screening with the EPDS, it is important to follow up screening with a clinical interview. Oates (2003) argues that cut-off points should not be used to diagnose PND; rather, a clinical interview is the gold standard and needs to follow screening to exclude other forms of mental illness. Researchers have found that women reject the label of depression as they believe that they are not depressed (Brown et al. 1994; Whitton et al. 1996).

2.3.1.4 Routine Screening

There is much debate in the literature about the routine screening of women for PND using the EPDS. In their book, *Perinatal Mental Health. A Guide to the Edinburgh Postnatal Depression Scale,* Cox and Holden (2003:26) oppose the *routine* screening of women for depression as they argue that it is both 'unnecessary' and 'intrusive'. Underpinning this belief is that health professionals who are in *frequent contact* with women can rely on their skills to determine if women are depressed or not. Although these skills are not described, it can be assumed that Cox and Holden (2003) are referring to the powers of observation and good interviewing skills. Oates (2003) challenges using the EPDS as a routine screening tool as it disregards the experience of the health professional in detecting depression. Furthermore, Oates (2003) argues that using the EPDS assumes that the health professionals, specifically general practitioners, would know how to treat PND effectively.

In summary, studies have identified that up to 67% of women were falsely diagnosed with depression following screening with the EPDS. The validation of EPDS is affected by the sample size and population, timing of screening, the presentation of EPDS to the mother, the cut-off scores used and importantly, whether or not the screening is followed with a clinical interview.

2.3.2 Beck Depression Inventory

The Beck Depression Inventory (BDI-I) (Appendix B) was developed by Beck and colleagues (1961) to screen for depression and to monitor the effectiveness of treatment for depression. BDI-I is a self-report measure with 21 questions with four potential responses for each question (scored 0–3). The total score identifies the severity of depression. For example, 1–10 is normal; 11–16 indicates a mild mood disturbance; 17–20 identifies borderline clinical depression; 21–30, moderate depression; 31–40, severe depression; and over 40 identifies extreme depression (Beck et al. 1961). The BDI-I differs from the EPDS as it assesses the cognition and motivation of individuals, not just the physiological symptoms (Sloan et al. 2002). The BDI-I and the EPDS are both based on the frequency of depressive symptoms.

A more recent version of BDI-I, BDI-II, was updated by Beck et al. (1996). The BDI-I and BDI-II are both self-report measures asking how people have felt over the past 2 weeks (Sharp and Lipsky 2002). The BDI-II was developed to more closely match the diagnosis of depressive disorders according to the DSM-IV-TR. The revised BDI has additional questions about stress, anxiety and isolation.

2.3.2.1 Critiques of the Beck Depression Inventory

The BDI-I has been critiqued for its poor sensitivity in detecting depression (Sloan et al. 2002). In their study of 319 anxious clients (174 females), Sloan and associates (2002) found that when they used the cut-off score of above 20 with BDI-I, over one third of the samples was misdiagnosed with depression. Furthermore, Sloan et al. (2002) recommended using the cut-off score of 23 on the BDI-I or score of 27 on the BDI-II to avoid diagnosing anxious clients with depression. They concluded that the BDI-I should not be used in isolation to diagnose depression.

Studies have also identified that the BDI-I has poor validity when it is used to detect antenatal depression (Sharp and Lipsky 2002) and PND (Beck and Gable 2000; Cox et al. 1987; Sloan et al. 2002). Furthermore, and not surprisingly, Cox et al. (1987) recommend using the EPDS instead of the BDI in the postpartum period for two reasons. First, BDI focuses on somatic symptoms of depression, which may be due to normal physiological changes after birth. Second, EPDS is a shorter screening scale as it consists of 10, instead of 21, questions.

2.3.3 Postpartum Depression Screening Scale

The Postpartum Depression Screening Scale (PDSS) was developed by Beck and Gable (2000, 2001, 2002) in the United States to specifically detect women at risk of developing PND. It is only available online (Kennedy et al. 2002). The PDSS is a 35-question, self-report instrument and asks how women have felt over the past 2 weeks (Beck and Gable 2001; Clemmens et al. 2004). Beck and Gable (2000) developed the PDSS from a sample of 525 mothers. The Likert-type scale rates questions from 1 (strongly disagree) to 5 (strongly agree), and the questions are exact quotes from Beck's qualitative studies (1992, 1993, 1996). The PDSS covers seven dimensions of PND: sleeping/eating disturbances (difficulty sleeping, loss of appetite); anxiety/insecurity (bodily sensations, loneliness, feeling overwhelmed); emotional lability (different emotional states); cognitive difficulties (ability to concentrate); loss of self (feeling abnormal); guilt/shame (sense of failure, guilt or shame); and suicidal ideation (threat to self) (Clemmens et al. 2004; Kennedy et al. 2002). A cut-off score of 80 indicates that women have significant symptoms of PND (Kennedy et al. 2002). The PDSS has items that are not on the EPDS, such as loss of control, loneliness, unrealness, irritability, fear of going crazy, obsessive thinking, difficulty in concentrating and loss of self (Beck and Gable 2002). The PDSS has been validated with Spanish-speaking women (Beck and Gable 2003).

2.3.3.1 Critiques of the Postpartum Depression Screening Scale

The PDSS has been criticised for being a lengthy screening tool (Buist et al. 2002). Also, the PDSS is a relatively new instrument and therefore few studies have examined its reliability and validity compared with other screening tools. Shakespeare (2001) asserts that the PDSS has minimal positive predictive value over the EPDS. Cox and Holden (2003) advise health professionals to use the EPDS instead of the BDI and PDSS as the EPDS is used throughout the world and would enable researchers to compare findings. Clemmens and colleagues (2004) validated the PDSS in a sub-analysis of data from 150 new mothers (75%) who participated in Beck and Gable's (2001) earlier study. All women completed the PDSS and had a DSM-IV diagnostic interview with a nurse psychotherapist. Data analysis focused on exploring the profiles of women regardless of whether or not they were diagnosed with PND (Clemmens et al. 2004). Eighteen of the 150 mothers were diagnosed with major PND, 18 were diagnosed with minor PND, and 104 were not depressed. The majority of women in the non-depressed group circled 1 ('strongly disagree') to questions across all seven dimensions. In contrast, most of the women diagnosed with minor or major depression circled 2 or 3 across these dimensions. Clemmens et al. (2004) concluded that PDSS is a reliable and valid instrument for screening women for PND and provided health professionals with details of the severity, frequency and intensity of depressive symptoms along a continuum ranging from not depressed to PND.

In summary, the screening tools have significant cut-off scores to detect women at risk of depression or PND. Screening is also used to expedite treatment (Evins et al. 2000; Georgiopoulos et al. 2001; Harvie 2004). Although screening tools are important for detecting PND, there are limitations when using them without a clinical interview as higher rates of depression have been reported (Busfield 1996; O'Hara and Swain 1996). Screening tools can also limit the interaction between the health professional and the woman. For example, Barker (1998) suggests that when a screening tool is used, the health visitor may focus on form filling rather than using their clinical skills and experience to detect depression. Another dilemma is that normal postnatal symptoms could be identified as depressive symptoms when the screening tool is used alone (Eberhard-Gran et al. 2001). Ideally, a clinical interview should follow screening to determine psychosocial stressors rather than solely relying on the screening tool to diagnose PND.

2.4   The Clinical Interview

Health professionals using a biopsychosocial model of health are more likely to use a clinical interview to diagnose psychiatric illnesses rather than relying on screening tools alone (Sommers-Flanagan and Sommers-Flanagan 2003). From a biomedical or psychiatric perspective, the primary aim of a clinical interview is to identify the appropriate diagnosis and treatment for an individual (Sommers-Flanagan and Sommers-Flanagan 2003). Table 2.2, *Aspects of the clinical interview*, draws on the biopsychosocial model of health as it addresses all of the components of the model. The clinical interview may include one or more of the following: a complete history, mental status examination, laboratory testing and the use of the DSM-IV-TR to rule out other mood disorders and to diagnose psychiatric illness (Lankin 2006). However, in the literature, there are different definitions of clinical interviewing. Some definitions reflect the imbalance of power between the interviewer and the interviewee where the interviewer asks the questions and the interviewee responds to the questions (Keates 2000; Shea 1998). A more comprehensive definition of clinical interviewing was proposed by Sommers-Flanagan and Sommers-Flanagan (2003:17) who defined clinical interviewing as a process by which 'the interviewer and client work together, to some extent, to establish and achieve mutually agreeable goals for the client'.

Table 2.2 Aspects of the clinical interview

Complete history
- Age, sex, marital status, medications, drug/alcohol use
- Previous psychiatric, medical and social history (from childhood to now)
- Chief complaint (mood, sleep, appetite, energy level, memory and concentration, loss of interest, suicidal ideation)

Mental status examination
- Appearance and behaviour (grooming, energy level, body language)
- Speech (loudness, speed, vocabulary, articulation)
- Mood and affect (mood is a sustained emotional state; affect is the patient's current emotional state)
- Thought form and content (logic and coherence)
- Assessment of thought content (abnormal preoccupations and obsessions, delusions, hallucinations, suicidal or homicidal ideation)
- Cognition (attention, concentration, orientation, memory, intellectual functioning)
- Insight and judgment (the patient's recognition of signs and symptoms and the impairment of judgment)

Laboratory testing
- Full blood count
- Thyroid function tests
- Depending upon symptoms – drug screen, blood alcohol, B12 and folate levels

DSM-IV-TR criteria
- To rule out other mood changes/disorders
- To determine specific psychiatric diagnosis

(Modified from Lankin 2006)

The American Psychiatric Association (2000) asserts the importance of using a clinical interview to identify symptoms of a major depressive episode. As a result, it has published a book, *The Clinical Interview Using DSM-IV-TR*, as a guideline to diagnostic interviewing. The authors Othmer and Othmer (2002) suggest four key components of interviewing – rapport (how the interviewer and patient relate); technique (methods used by the interviewer to develop rapport and obtain information); mental status (mood, energy level, perception and content of thinking); and diagnosis. Sommers-Flanagan and Sommers-Flanagan (2003) broaden this perspective to include individual social support network (interviewing others to obtain accurate information, particularly if the individual lacks the insight to identify his or her symptoms) and physical examination (gathering information from other health professionals and/or laboratory findings).

The following quote by Othmer and Othmer (2002:9) highlights the medical model's perception of individuals with mental illnesses as having 'weaknesses' or flaws in their personalities. The quote also identifies the aim of the clinical interview to obtain an 'appropriate and accurate diagnosis':

> The more the interviewer learns about the patient's strengths, weaknesses, and suffering, the better able she is to render an appropriate and accurate diagnosis. The more experienced she is and the more she knows about the disorder, stressors, and coping skills, the better she can assess them.

An important point is noted in the aforementioned quote that health professionals' knowledge and experience of mental illnesses affect the accuracy of the diagnoses. Although this may be important from a medical or psychiatric perspective, health professionals using a clinical interview would be more likely to focus on the individual's problems or symptoms, which may assist them to resolve identified problems (Sommers-Flanagan and Sommers-Flanagan 2003). Thus, this approach places more emphasis on the identification of the individual's problems and a lesser emphasis on the establishment of a psychiatric diagnosis.

2.4.1 From Screening to Diagnosis

One of the challenges faced by health professionals is the early detection of depressive symptoms when women hide their distress. Women with PND often mask their symptoms of depression, making diagnosis more difficult as they feel ashamed of being labelled 'bad mothers' (Buist 1996; Maushart 1997; Buultjens and Liamputtong 2007). Other women fear their babies will be taken away if they admit to being depressed (Brown et al. 1994). Furthermore, women with PND often suffer in silence and are reluctant to seek help (Beck and Gable 2001; McIntosh 1993; Shakespeare 2001).

The leap from screening to diagnosis is important for the argument in our book that women are often not given the opportunity to discuss psychosocial factors that contribute to their emotional health when only screening tools are used. The definition of PND is broad and confusing, therefore posing challenges in terms of diagnosis. Postnatal depression is often confused with other mood disorders or is not detected at all (Buist 1996; National Health and Medical Research Council 2000). Postnatal depression is a generic term covering a wide range of mild to severe disorders (Oates 2003) and is sometimes used when women develop chronic depression (Shakespeare 2001) and antenatal depression (Milgrom et al. 1999). Recently, and adding to the confusion with the definition of PND, the term 'perinatal depression' has been used to classify both antenatal and postnatal depression (Beyond Blue 2010).

Postnatal depression is difficult to diagnose close to delivery as women often experience sadness, exhaustion, loss of self-esteem and both sleep and appetite disturbances in the postpartum period (Beck and Gable 2001). In clinical practice, women often do not develop symptoms of PND within 4 weeks of childbirth to meet the DSM-IV criteria for diagnosis (Milgrom et al. 1999). Buist (1996) contends that women with PND are often not diagnosed after their first baby but rather following subsequent pregnancies due to misdiagnosis or failure to diagnose.

There is much debate about the use of antenatal screening tools to prevent PND (Priest et al. 2006). The Postpartum Depression Predictors Inventory (Beck 2002c) for use in the antenatal and postnatal period to detect women at risk of developing PND is awaiting validation trials.

2.5 Chapter Summary

In this chapter, we have critiqued three screening tools used to identify women at risk of developing PND – the Edinburgh Postnatal Depression Scale, the Beck Depression Inventory and the Postpartum Depression Screening Scale. The most commonly used screening tool, the Edinburgh Postnatal Depression Screening Scale, was the main focus of the chapter. The validity of the Edinburgh Postnatal Depression Scale is dependent upon the timing of assessment, cut-off scores used, the presentation of the tool to the mother, the sample population and recruitment strategies used, and whether or not EPDS was followed by a clinical interview to confirm diagnosis. The main concern with all of these screening tools is that they are purely screening and not diagnostic tools.

We discussed the historical development of PND as a category of mental illness that evolved from the DSM, ICD-10 and the Research Diagnostic Criteria. The American Psychiatric Association's (2000) DSM-IV-TR criteria for diagnosing PND were discussed with other mood disorders. Whilst the DSM-IV-TR categories are helpful for providing consistency in psychiatric diagnoses, there are also limitations as women's symptoms are reduced into distinct categories rather than identifying individual stressors that contribute to depressive symptoms. The diagnosis of PND requires communication between the mother and the health professional. The diagnosis of PND may also be affected by the experience and knowledge of the health professional in identifying the symptoms of PND. The clinical interview provides an apportunity for health professionals to explore the psychosocial factors contributing to PND, and it provides a bridge between screening and diagnosis.

In the next chapter, we will discuss the importance of using a biopsychosocial approach when treating women for PND. We will also explore the differences between the biomedical and sociological models in their understanding and treatment of PND.

References

American Psychiatric Association. (1952). *Diagnostic and statistical manual of mental disorders, DSM-I* (1st ed.). Washington, DC: American Psychiatric Press.
American Psychiatric Association. (1968). *Diagnostic and statistical manual of mental disorders, DSM-II* (2nd ed.). Washington, DC: American Psychiatric Press.
American Psychiatric Association. (1980). *Diagnostic and statistical manual of mental disorders, DSM III* (3rd ed.). Washington, DC: American Psychiatric Press.
American Psychiatric Association. (1987). *Diagnostic and statistical manual of mental disorders, DSM III-R* (3 revisedth ed.). Washington, DC: American Psychiatric Press.
American Psychiatric Association. (1994). *Diagnostic and statistical manual of mental disorders, DSM-IV* (4th ed.). Washington, DC: American Psychiatric Press.
American Psychiatric Association. (2000). *Diagnostic and statistical manual of mental disorders, text revision. DSM-IV-TR* (4 revisedth ed.). Washington, DC: American Psychiatric Press.
Austin, M. P. (2003). Psychosocial assessment and management of depression and anxiety in pregnancy. Key aspects of antenatal care for general practice. *Australian Family Physician, 32*(3), 119–126.

Austin, M. P., & Lumley, J. (2003). Antenatal screening for postnatal depression: A systematic review. *Acta Psychiatrica Scandinavia, 107*(1), 10–17.

Barker, W. (1998). Let's trust our instincts. *Community Practitioner, 71*, 305.

Beck, C. (1992). The lived experience of postpartum depression: A phenomenological study. *Nursing Research, 41*(3), 166–170.

Beck, C. T. (1993). Teetering on the edge: A substantive theory of postpartum depression. *Nursing Research, 42*, 42–48.

Beck, C. T. (1996). Postpartum depressed mothers' experiences interacting with their children. *Nursing Research, 45*, 98–104.

Beck, C. (1999). Postpartum depression: Stopping the thief that steals motherhood. *AWHONN Lifelines, 3*(4), 41–44.

Beck, C. T. (2002a). Theoretical perspectives of postpartum depression and their treatment implications. *The American Journal of Maternal/Child Nursing, 27*(5), 282–287.

Beck, C. T. (2002b). Revision of the Postpartum Depression Predictors Inventory. *Journal of Obstetric, Gynecologic and Neonatal Nursing, 31*, 391–402.

Beck, C., & Gable, R. K. (2000). Postpartum depression screening scale: Development and psychometric Testing. *Nursing Research, 49*(5), 272–282.

Beck, C., & Gable, R. K. (2001). Further validation of the postpartum depression screening scale. *Nursing Research, 50*(3), 155–164.

Beck, C. T., & Gable, R. K. (2002). *The postpartum depression screening scale manual.* Los Angeles: Webster Psychological Association.

Beck, C. T., & Gable, R. K. (2003). Postpartum depression screening scale: Spanish version. *Nursing Research, 52*(5), 296–306.

Beck, A. T., Ward, C. H., Mendelson, M., Mock, J., & Erbaugh, J. (1961). An inventory for measuring depression. *Archives of General Psychiatry, 4*, 561–571.

Beck, A., Steer, R., & Brown, G. (1996). *BDI-II manual.* San Antonio: The Psychological Corporation.

Beyond Blue. (2010). What is postnatal depression? http://www.beyondblue.org.au/index.aspx?link_id=94. Accessed 28 May 2010.

Boyce, P., Stubbs, J., & Todd, A. (1993). The Edinburgh postnatal depression scale: Validation for an Australian sample. *Australian and New Zealand Journal of Psychiatry, 27*, 472–476.

Brown, G. W., & Harris, T. (1978). *Social origins of depression. A study of psychiatric disorder in women.* London: Tavistock Publications Limited.

Brown, G. W., & Harris, T. O. (2001). *Life events and illness.* New York: Guilford Press.

Brown, S., Lumley, J., Small, R., & Astbury, J. (1994). *Missing voices. The experience of motherhood.* Melbourne: Oxford University Press.

Brown, G. W., Harris, T. O., & Hepworth, C. (1995). Loss, humiliation and entrapment among women developing depression: A patient and non-patient comparison. *Psychological Medicine, 25*(1), 7–22.

Buist, A. (1996). *Psychiatric disorders associated with childbirth.* Sydney: McGraw-Hill.

Buist, A. (2002). Mental health in pregnancy: The sleeping giant. *Australasian Psychiatry, 10*(3), 203–206.

Buist, A., Barnett, B., Milgrom, J., Pope, S., Condon, J. T., Ellwood, D. A., et al. (2002). To screen or not to screen- that is the question in perinatal depression. *Medical Journal of Australia, 177*(7 October), S101–S105.

Busfield, J. (1996). *Men, women and madness. Understanding gender and mental disorder.* London: MacMillan.

Buultjens, M., & Liamputtong, P. (2007). When giving life starts to take the life out of you: Women's experiences of depression after childbirth. *Midwifery, 23*, 77–91.

Clemmens, D., Driscoll, J. W., & Beck, C. T. (2004). Postpartum depression as profiled through the depression screening scale. *The American Journal of Maternal/Child Nursing, 29*(3), 180–185. May/June.

Cox, J. L., & Holden, J. (2003). *Perinatal mental health. A Guide to the Edinburgh Postnatal Depression Scale (EPDS).* London: Gaskell.

Cox, J., Holden, J., & Sagovsky, R. (1987). Detection of postnatal depression: Development of the 10 item Edinburgh Postnatal Depression Scale. *British Journal of Psychiatry, 150*, 782–786.

Eaker, E. D. (2005). Social support and physical health: Understanding the health consequences of relationships. *American Journal of Epidemiology, 161*(3), 297–298.

Eberhard-Gran, M., Eskild, A., Tambs, K., Opjordsmoen, S., & Samuelsen, S. O. (2001). Review of validation studies of the Edinburgh Postnatal Depression Scale. *Acta Psychiatrica Scandinavica, 104*(4), 243–249.

Eriksen, K., & Kress, V. E. (2005). *Beyond the DSM story*. Thousand Oaks: Sage.

Evins, G. G., Theofrastous, J. P., & Galvin, S. L. (2000). Postpartum depression: A comparison of screening and routine clinical evaluation. *American Journal of Obstetrics & Gynecology, 182*, 1080–1082.

Fettling, L. (2002). *Postnatal depression. A practical guide for Australian families*. Melbourne: IP Communications.

Georgiopoulos, A. M., Bryan, T. L., Wollan, P., & Yawn, B. P. (2001). Routine screening for postpartum depression. *Journal of Family Practice, 50*, 117–122.

Goldberg, D. P. (1972). *The detection of psychiatric illness by questionnaire (Maudsley Monographs*, Vol. 21). Oxford: Oxford University Press.

Goldberg, D. P., Cooper, B., Eastwood, M. R., Kedward, H. B., & Shepherd, M. (1970). A standardised psychiatric interview for use in community surveys. *British Journal of Preventive and Social Medicine, 24*, 18–23.

Harris, T. (2001). Recent developments in understanding the psychosocial aspects of depression. *British Medical Bulletin, 57*, 17–32.

Harris, T. (2003). Book review. Postnatal depression: Facing the paradox of loss, happiness and motherhood. *Journal of Child Psychology and Psychiatry, 44*(6), 930.

Harvie, J. (2004, March 11). Screening program raises awareness. *Sydney Morning Herald*, p. 2.

Keates, D. M. (2000). *Interviewing: A practical guide for students and professionals*. Buckingham, England, Open University Press.

Kennedy, H. P., Beck, C., & Driscoll, J. W. (2002). A light in the fog: Caring for women with postpartum depression. *Journal of Midwifery and Women's Health, 47*(5), 318–330.

Lankin, K. (2006). Mental status exam and diagnostic modalitites. http://wwwbrooksidepress.org/Products/OperationalMedicine/Data/operationalmed/. Accessed 5 July 2006.

Marcé Society. (2006). http://www.marcesociety.com/home.php3. Accessed 5 July 2006.

Maushart, S. (1997). *The mask of motherhood*. Sydney: Random House.

Mauthner, N. S. (2002). *The darkest days of my life. Stories of postpartum depression*. Cambridge: Harvard University Press.

McIntosh, J. (1993). Postpartum depression: women's help-seeking behaviour and perceptions of cause. *Journal of Advanced Nursing, 18*, 178–184.

Meier, A. (1979). The research diagnostic criteria: historical background, development, validity, and reliability. *Canadian Journal of Psychiatry, 24*(2): 167–178.

Milgrom, J., Martin, P. R., & Negri, L. M. (1999). *Treating postnatal depression. A psychological approach for health care practitioners*. Chichester: Wiley.

National Health and Medical Research Council. (2000). Postnatal depression. A systematic review of published scientific literature to 1999. http://www.nhmrc.gov.au/publications/synopses/wh29syn.htm.Accessed 12 June 2007.

Oakley, A. (1980). *Women confined. Towards a sociology of childbirth*. Oxford: Martin Robinson.

Oates, M. R. (2003). Postnatal depression and screening: Too broad a sweep? *British Journal of General Practice, 53*, 596–597. August.

O'Hara, M. W., & Swain, A. M. (1996). Rates and risk of postpartum depression- a meta-analysis. *International Review of Psychiatry, 8*, 37–54.

O'Hara, M. W., Schlechte, J. A., & Lewis, D. A. (1991). Psychiatric disorders in the postpartum period. *BC Medical Journal, 47*(2), 100–102.

Othmer, E., & Othmer, S. C. (2002). *The clinical interview using DSM-IV-TR: Vol. 1. Fundamentals*. Washington, DC: American Psychiatric Publishing.

Paris, R., & Dubus, N. (2005). Staying connected while nurturing and infant: A challenge of new motherhood. *Family Relations, 54*, 72–83.

Pilgrim, D., & Bentall, R. (1999). The medicalisation of misery: A critical realist analysis of the concept of depression. *Journal of Mental Health, 69*, 135–138.

Pitt, B. (1968). "Atypical" depression following childbirth. *British Journal of Psychiatry, 114*, 1325–1335.

Priest, S. R., Austin, M., & Sullivan, E. A. (2006). Antenatal psychosocial screening for prevention of antenatal and postnatal anxiety and depression. *Cochrane Database for Systematic Reviews, 1*, No page number.

Ray, K. L., & Hodnett, E. D. (2006). Caregiver support for postpartum depression. *Cochrane Database for Systematic Reviews, 1*, No page number.

Robins, L., Helzer, J., Cottler, L., & Goldring, E. (1989). *NIMH Diagnostic Interview Schedule.* Version 3 revised.

Robins, L.N, Helzer, J.E., Croughan, J., & Ratcliffe, S (1981). National Institute of Mental Health Diagnostic Interview Schedule. Archives of General Psychiatry, (38), 381–390

Ryan, D., & Kostaras, X. (2005). Psychiatric disorders in the postpartum period. *British Columbia Medical Journal, 47*(2), 100–103.

Seligman, M. E. (1975). *Helplessness. On depression, development, and death.* San Francisco: W.H. Freeman and Company.

Shakespeare, J. (2001). Evaluation of screening for postnatal depression against the NSC handbook criteria. Prepared for a working party. www.nelh.nhs.uk/screening/adult_pps/postnatal_depression.html. Accessed July 2002.

Sharp, L. K., & Lipsky, M. S. (2002). Depression across the lifespan: A review of measures for use in primary care setttings. *American Family Physician, 66*(6), 1001–1008.

Shea, S. C. (1998). *Psychiatric interviewing: The art of understanding.* Philadelphia, Saunders.

Sloan, D. M., Marx, B. P., Bradley, M. M., Strauss, C. C., Lang, P. I., & Cuthbert, B. C. (2002). Examining the high-end specificity of the Beck depression inventory using an anxiety sample. *Cognitive Therapy and Research, 26*(6), 719–727.

Sommers-Flanagan, J., & Sommers-Flanagan, R. (2003). *Clinical interviewing* (3rd ed.). New Jersey: Wiley.

Spitzer, R., Endicott, J., & Robins, E. (1975). *Research Diagnostic Criteria. Instrument No. 58.* New York: New York State Psychiatric Institute.

Spitzer, R. L., Endicott, J., & Robins, E. (1978). Research diagnostic criteria: Rationale and reliability. *Archives of General Psychiatry, 35*, 773–782.

Spitzer, R. L., Williams, J. B. W., & Skodol, A. E. (1983). *International perspectives on DSM-III.* Washington, DC: American Psychiatric Press.

Whitton, A., Warner, R., & Appleby, L. (1996). The pathway to care in post-natal depression: Women's attitudes to post-natal depression and its treatment. *British Journal of General Practice, 46*, 427–428.

WHO. (1992). *The ICD-10 classification of mental and behavioural disorders. Clinical descriptions and diagnostic guidelines.* Geneva: World Health Organization.

WHO. (2000). *Women's mental health. An evidenced based review.* Geneva: WHO.

Wickberg, B., & Hwang, C. (1996). The Edinburgh postnatal depression scale: Validation on a Swedish community sample. *Acta Psychiatrica Scandinavica, 94*(3), 181–184.

Williams, J. B., & Spitzer, R. L. (1982). Research diagnostic criteria and DSM-III: an annotated comparison. *Archives of General Psychiatry 39*(11).

Wisner, K. L., Parry, B. L., & Piontek, C. M. (2002). Postpartum Depression. *The New England Journal of Medicine, 347*(3), 194–199.

World Health Organization (2006). International Classification of Diseases (ICD) http://www.who.int/classifications/icd/en/ Accessed July 2006.

Chapter 3
Biopsychosocial Theories and Treatment Options for Postnatal Depression

Our aim in this chapter is to provide a broad theoretical understanding of PND. The study on which this book is based aimed to explore how women and their partners understand and resolve PND. The emphasis will be placed on the psycho-social factors in the development and resolution of PND. In this chapter, we will examine the differences between the biomedical and sociological models in their understanding and treatment of PND. As previously discussed, the biomedical model has been the dominant model in the literature investigating PND (Beck 2002), but this model only partially explains the illness. In this chapter, we argue that a biopsychosocial approach is needed to fully understand PND because using only the biomedical model neglects the personal, social and cultural context of women's experiences.

The first section, 'The biopsychosocial model', will provide a broad overview of the model proposed by Engel in 1977. The biopsychosocial model is a holistic approach to health care and has three dimensions – biological, psychological and sociological components. Two existing models relating to PND (Brown and Harris 1978; Milgrom et al. 1999) will also be discussed.

In the second section, 'Biological theories and treatments of PND', we will discuss the biomedical model's theories about the development of PND and their treatment strategies. The traditional medical understanding of PND as a hormonal and physiological problem needing treatment will be discussed with the various pharmacological interventions.

In the third section, 'Psychosocial theories and treatments', we will explore the sociological model's understanding of PND such as gender, significant life events and the lack of support, as it acknowledges the personal and social factors that contribute to PND. Based on this approach, the treatment of PND would focus on increasing women's support network and their self-esteem. The main focus of this section will be the importance of social support for women's emotional well-being, as it was identified as a major gap in the literature.

C. Westall and P. Liamputtong, *Motherhood and Postnatal Depression: Narratives of Women and Their Partners*, DOI 10.1007/978-94-007-1694-0_3,
© Springer Science+Business Media B.V. 2011

3.1   The Biopsychosocial Model

In psychiatry, the biopsychosocial model is the overriding paradigm used for the assessment and management of mental illnesses (Stocky 1992). The biopsychosocial model acknowledges the dynamic nature of the biological, psychological and social dimensions of health and illness (Engel 1977). George Engel (1977) developed the biopsychosocial model to encompass the missing dimensions of the biomedical model and to provide a holistic approach to health care. He challenged the biomedical model for its reductionism, for mind-body dualism and for ignoring the broader social and cultural influences affecting the health of individuals . In contrast, the biopsycho-social model provides a conceptual framework for physicians to use in clinical practice and enables physicians to become more informed about the psychosocial factors that contribute to ill-health (Engel 1977). For example, physicians using the biopsycho-social model could improve the treatment of depression by tailoring it specifically to the individual's needs (Novack 2003).

The biopsychosocial model is a way of understanding suffering, disease and illness from the molecular to societal levels (Borrell-Carrio et al. 2004; Ferrer et al. 2005; see Fig. 3.1).

In Fig. 3.1, each level in the hierarchy represents a dynamic whole and causes changes within the system (Engel 1977). Originally, Engel (1977) proposed the levels in the hierarchy using an example of an individual with myocardial damage. We have adapted the levels in the hierarchy to encompass the range of biopsychoso-cial factors that influence the emotional well-being of women with PND. For exam-ple, even though the pathological process at the cellular or organ level could be resolved (for example with antidepressants), sometimes psychosocial disturbances continue, such as the lack of support from others.

Hanson (2007) provides a simplistic view of Engel's (1977) biopsychosocial model, as represented in Fig. 3.2. The biological or sensory component refers to the medical or physical aspects of depression, such as fatigue or anxiety. The psycho-logical factors include three components – the mental (cognitive awareness of depres-sion); emotional (any emotional state, such as depression); and behavioural aspects (what you do about the depressive symptoms). The social factors refer to the interac-tions between individuals that influence the experience of depression. For example, when an individual is emotionally well, the elements of the biopsychosocial model are all in harmony with one another. Disharmony occurs when depression (sensory) results in negative emotional reactions (emotional), isolation from others (social), decreased self-worth (mental) and loss of motivation (behavioural) (Hanson 2007).

3.1.1   Previous Models Relating to PND

Originally, a social model for depression in women was proposed by two academic sociologists, Brown and Harris (1978), in their book, *Social Origins of Depression: A study of psychiatric disorder in women*. They performed the first in-depth study

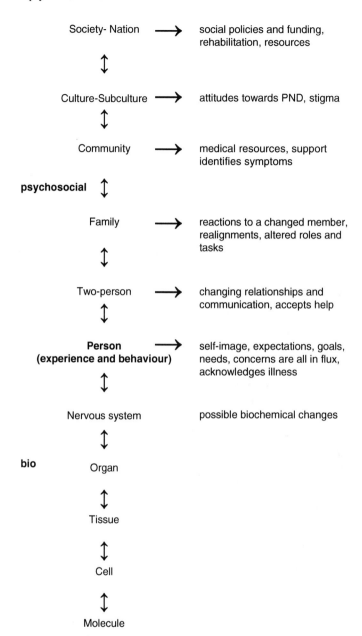

Fig. 3.1 Levels of Influence on individual experiences of PND (Modified from Engel 1980; Drew 2003)

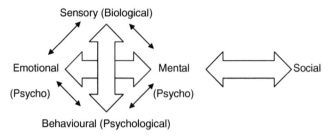

Fig. 3.2 Biopsychosocial interactions (Modified from Hanson 2007)

investigating the role of social factors in depression. Brown and Harris (1978) chal-lenged biological, hormonal and reproductive explanations for depression. Their social model for depression has three main elements: provoking elements or severe life events, such as important losses and disappointments or major difficulties last-ing for more than 2 years; vulnerability factors, such as a non-confiding marriage; and maintaining factors, such as the presence of an anxiety disorder. Brown and Harris (1978) identified four vulnerability factors that increased women's risk of developing depression – parental loss before the age of 17, particularly the loss of a mother before the age of 11; having three or more children younger than 14 at home; a non-confiding marriage; and the lack of full or part-time employment.

In more recent times, psychologists Milgrom and colleagues (1999) built on the social model of depression proposed by Brown and Harris (1978) and created the biopsychosocial model specifically for women with PND. Their model was developed from the empirical literature and from their own clinical experience. However, Milgrom et al. (1999, p.25) admitted their own model was 'speculative and incom-plete' as there were limited methodologically sound studies in the literature. These models were included as they highlight the importance of identifying the psychosocial factors contributing to depression and PND. These factors would influence the specific treatment required for the individual.

3.2   The Importance of Treatment

Postnatal depression and depression are treated the same way; the only difference is that women with PND have the added burden of caring for their children (Buist et al. 2002). A biopsychosocial approach is needed to provide a holistic approach to treatment. The following quote by Fullager and Gattuso (2002: 3) high-lights the importance of using a biopsychosocial approach when treating women with PND:

> The emphasis on biomedical explanations and treatments means that the more complex social and cultural processes shaping women's experiences of depression, emotional well-being and mental illness remain poorly recognized.

The treatment of PND also depends upon the severity of symptoms (Kwok 2003; National Health and Medical Research Council 2000). Mild to moderate cases of PND can be treated with a range of treatments, such as complementary therapies, antidepressant medication, group or individual counselling and cognitive behavioural therapy (CBT) (Kwok 2003). More severe cases of PND may require a combination of treatments, such as psychotherapy and antidepressant medication (National Health and Medical Research Council 2000). Women may require admission to a psychiatric hospital or a mother-baby unit if treatments are ineffective or if women are at risk of hurting themselves or their infants. Regardless of the severity of PND, it is important to determine if there is a risk of infanticide or suicide.

There are also personal costs if depression remains untreated or is treated incorrectly. In severe cases, people may lose the ability to function, work or care for themselves (American Psychiatric Association 2000). Ongoing depression can have a profound effect on all aspects of an individual's being, such as their feelings, thoughts, emotions, functioning and relationships. The importance of an individual's mental health for their employment, relationships and self-esteem are well-documented. The World Health Organization (2001) discusses the importance of social and emotional well-being for an individual's mental health:

> [Mental health] is a state of emotional and social well-being in which the individual realises his or her own abilities, can cope with the normal stresses of life, can work productively or fruitfully, and is able to make a contribution to his or her community (WHO website).

Therefore, mental health is important for individuals to be able to cope with stress, for their relationships with others and for their contribution to society.

3.2.1 Biological Theories and Treatments

The medical model has been the dominant model in managing PND (Beck 2002) and defines depression as a hormonal and physiological problem associated with reproduction (Borrell-Carrio et al. 2004; Patel 2001). A plethora of research has attempted to find the biological cause for depression. Despite these numerous studies, the findings remain inconclusive as to the specific biochemical and hormonal changes responsible for the development of PND (Harmer et al. 2003; Lawrie et al. 2003; Morrow et al. 2008). Hormonal changes have been investigated in depressed individuals, such as progesterone, oestrogen, cortisone, endorphins, oxytocin and prolactin levels (Gordon et al. 1980; Smith et al. 1989; Wieck et al. 1991; Wisner et al. 2002). Other researchers have explored the role of biochemical changes in the development of depression by assessing levels of serotonin (5-hydroxytryptamine or 5-HT) and norepinephrine (Cleare et al. 1997; Lawrie et al. 2003).

Biochemical changes can also occur with stress. Anand and Charney (2000) have found that levels of norepinephrine can be depleted with chronic stress, thereby contributing to depressive symptoms. The hypothalamic-pituitary-adrenal (HPA) axis is thought to be activated by both stress and depression (Cacioppo 1994; Oshimer et al. 2001) and is crucial for regulating the severity of disease (Harbuz 2002).

According to Leonard (2001), stress is a major contributing factor to the development of depression and is responsible for changes in the immune, endocrine and norepinephrine systems. This finding suggests that treating individuals when they are stressed could prevent the development of depression.

3.2.1.1 Pharmacological Interventions

Predominantly, the medical model uses pharmacological treatments for women with PND (Appleby et al. 1997). However, this focus on the biological symptoms means that the psychosocial factors that could be contributing to PND are ignored. Antidepressant medication targets different neurotransmitters in the brain. For example, the tricyclic antidepressants and monoamine oxidase inhibitors (MAOI's) increase the levels of norepinephrine (noradrenaline) in the brain (Seligman and Rosenhan 1998). In contrast, the selective serotonin reuptake inhibitors (SSRI's) increase serotonin levels in the brain (Seligman and Rosenhan 1998). However, it is not known which chemical in the brain is deficient before commencing treatment. It is also not known how these biochemical changes improve the depressed mood of individuals. Harmer and colleagues (2003: 990) highlight this point:

> Antidepressants that increase serotonin or norepinephrine in the brain are effective in treating depression, but there is no neuropsychological account of how these changes relieve depressive states.

The Victorian Drug Usage Advisory Committee (2003: 155) recommends that if patients failed to respond to antidepressants, they should be referred to a psychiatrist and the following questions should be asked:

- Is the diagnosis correct?
- Has the patient been taking their medication regularly?
- Have possible underlying physical causes been identified and treated?
- Have the dosage and duration of administration of the drug been adequate?
- Have relevant psychosocial or personality factors been addressed?
- Has alcohol or drug use been addressed?
- Could an interacting drug be compromising response?
- Is the patient metabolising the drug rapidly?

These recommendations put forward by the Victorian Drug Usage Advisory Committee (2003) highlight the range of biopsychosocial factors that affect the efficacy of treatment with antidepressant medication. For antidepressant medication to be effective, the Victorian Drug Usage Advisory Committee (2003) advises that health professionals address the psychosocial factors, and not just the physical causes of depression.

There are concerns about the safety of antidepressant medication. The United States Food and Drug Administration (FDA) (2005) have issued a warning that antidepressant medication can increase the risk of suicidal behaviour in adults.

They advise health professionals to closely observe adults who are prescribed antidepressants for worsening of depressive symptoms and for suicidal behaviour, particularly at the beginning of treatment or when the doses are increased or decreased. Other treatments such as electroconvulsive therapy (ECT) or Lithium may also be considered (Victorian Drug Usage Advisory Committee 2003).

3.2.2 Psychosocial Theories and Treatments

The sociological model acknowledges the biological factors that impact on emotional well-being (Raeburn and Rootman 1989), but places more emphasis on the personal and social factors that contribute to depressive symptoms (WHO 2000). In Engel's (1977) biopsychosocial model, the 'psychological' refers to the relationship between the individual and their biological makeup, and the 'social' refers to the individual's interactions with others and the broader community. The 'psychosocial' is discussed together as we contend that the psychological and social factors are intertwined.

Numerous researchers have identified that psychosocial factors play a major role in the development of depression (Brown et al. 1986; Finlay-Jones 1989; Brown 1998; Buist 2006; Kinard 1990) and therefore cannot be explained by the medical model alone. Some of the psychosocial factors that can affect the emotional well-being of women include relationship difficulties (Eriksen and Kress 2005), poverty, social disadvantage, social class (WHO 2000), poor social support, past abuse (Buist 2006), low self-esteem, infant temperament and unrealistic expectations of motherhood (Milgrom et al. 1999).

Based on a psychosocial approach, the treatment of PND would aim to increase women's support network, improve their self-esteem, provide assistance with infant behaviour and reduce women's expectations of themselves. Other psychosocial treatments used for women with PND include individual counselling, group therapy, cognitive behavioural therapy and interpersonal psychotherapy (Milgrom et al. 1999). Furthermore, feminist theorists, Creedy and Shochet (1996), discuss the importance of identifying the triggers for PND, providing debriefing and encouraging women to talk about their roles as mothers to improve their emotional well-being. Other treatments may include increasing support to women after the birth, addressing violence, discussing past issues and assisting women with financial difficulties.

3.2.2.1 Gender and Depression

The World Health Organization (2000) asserts that women's emotional well-being needs to be examined within the social model of health, as gender is an important determinant of health affecting employment, income and socio-economic status.

The following quote by the WHO (2000: 15) highlights areas where women may be socially disadvantaged:

> It is vital, therefore, that women's health in general and women's mental health in particular, are examined within a social model which gives an account of the physical and mental health effects of common life stressors and events that disproportionately experienced by women. Clearly this cannot be confined to childbearing and reproductive events but must also include the impact of poverty, single parenthood, the 'double' shift of paid (often low paid) and unpaid work, employment status, lower wages, discrimination, physical, emotional and sexual violence and the psychological costs of childcare and other forms of caring work.

Women are twice as likely as men to develop depression, particularly in the child-bearing years (Austin and Lumley 2003; Busfield 1996; Sagud et al. 2002). Importantly, women will be depressed for a longer period of time than men and are more likely to need treatment for their depression (Austin and Lumley 2003). Researchers have attempted to explain gender differences in the rates of depression in relation to biological and physiological changes associated with reproduction (Davar 1999). However, gender differences in the rates of depression have not been adequately addressed (Bebbington 1998). Other researchers have explained the women's vulnerability to depression in terms of childbirth events and different psychosocial stresses for women (Burrows and Norman 2001), such as the lack of support and changes in work or financial circumstances around the time of the birth (Beck 1999; Brown and Harris 1978).

3.2.2.2 Significant Life Events

Pregnancy, childbirth and motherhood are significant life events in themselves. In the literature, significant life events have been linked to the onset of depressive symptoms (Brown 1998; Brown and Harris 1978; Brown et al. 1995; Harris 2001; Kendler et al. 2002, 2000; Morriss and Morriss 2000; Nazroo et al. 1997). Significant life events stem from some form of loss (Brown 1998). Brown and Harris (1978) were the first to acknowledge the role of significant life events in depression. They recruited a random sample of 154 untreated and treated depressed women aged 18–65 years from the Outer Hebrides, in Scotland and found that over half of the women had a significant life event contributing to depression. In their study, the significant life events women experienced were related to their employment, family role, health of self or family member, place of residence and the amount of contact with close relatives or family members. From their study, Brown and Harris (1978) identified that women who experienced two or more severe life events were more likely to experience depression. In congruence with the findings by Brown and Harris (1978), other researchers have found that the personal impact of the life event is influenced by the duration of the event and an individual's past and current social environment (Morriss and Morriss 2000). Brown (1998) found that it was the impact of the loss, rather than the event itself, that contributed to depression. For example, individuals with negative perceptions of life events were more likely to experience depression (Morriss and Morriss 2000).

3.2.2.3   Postnatal Depression in Different Regions and Cultures

The majority of qualitative studies have focused on women's experiences of PND in different countries, such as the United States (Beck 1992; 1993; 1996; Mauthner, 2002; Wood et al. 1997), Canada (Berggren-Clive 1998; Morrow et al. 2008), Hong Kong (Chan et al. 2002; Chan and Levy 2004), Laos (Stewart and Jambunathan 1996), Taiwan (Huang, and Mathers 2001), Australia (Nahas and Amasheh 1999; Nahas et al. 1999) and the United Kingdom (Mauthner 1999; 2002a, b). Stewart and Jambunathan (1996) found that cultural beliefs and practices of Hmong women helped their emotional well-being in the postpartum period. Some of the cultural practices included receiving support from partners and others and the 30-day rest period after the birth. On the other hand, Huang and Mathers (2001) found no difference in the rates of PND in their comparative study of women in the United Kingdom and Taiwan. They explained similar rates of depression in the two samples of women as a result of the modernisation of Taiwanese society and less women having a 30-day confinement after the birth. In a more recent study, Morrow and associates (2008) utilised an ethnographic narrative approach to explore immigrant women's experiences of postpartum depression in Canada. There were three groups of first generation Punjabi-speaking, Cantonese-speaking and Mandarin-speaking women. They found that women's narratives revealed the critical importance of the sociocultural context of childbirth in understanding postpartum depression. However, all of these studies lack the partners' perspectives of PND.

3.2.2.4   The Importance of Social Support

The terms 'social support' and 'support' are used interchangeably throughout this book as support requires some form of interaction with another human being. There is a scant amount of literature investigating the types of support women require in early motherhood to prevent and reduce depressive symptoms (Borjesson et al. 2004; Ray and Hodnett 2006). The importance of support from the partner is highlighted in the following quote by Ray and Hodnett (2006):

> Women with postpartum (postnatal) depression who are supported by caregivers are less likely to remain depressed, although the most effective support from caregivers remains unknown (no page number).

There is evidence in the literature that social support is important for an individual's self-esteem and sense of competence (Borjesson et al. 2004; Kitamura et al. 1999; Oakley 1992; Ray and Hodnett 2006). Social support can provide a buffer from stressful life events (Brown and Harris 1978) and can protect individuals from disease and early death (Eaker 2005). Support is important for women's emotional well-being because they need to feel connected to the broader social milieu to be able to feel accepted and understood by others. Mauthner (2002a, b: 131) highlights this point:

> Though the importance of strong, mutual relationships cannot be underestimated, the creation of an accepting, understanding, and non-judgmental broader cultural context in

which women can speak their feelings of ambivalence and depression without shame or stigma is equally critical.

Several researchers have identified that social support is the most important variable to consider when investigating PND (Kinard 1990; Ray and Hodnett 2006), as the lack of social support has been linked to depression and PND (Beck 1998; Borjesson et al. 2004; Brugha 1995; Gottlieb and Mendelson 1995; Kitzinger 1992; Mauthner 1999, 2002a, b; Ray and Hodnett 2006; Ugarriza 2002; WHO 2000; Wood et al. 1997). In an Australian study, Brown and colleagues (1994) interviewed 60 women who were depressed to explore what factors they attributed to their depression. Of these women, ten identified lack of support as the main association with depression, nine reported isolation, eight related it to tiredness and seven identified illness or death of a loved one as a significant factor. Furthermore, only one woman associated her depression with hormonal changes (Brown et al. 1994).

Social support has been defined in many ways. The definition by Brown (1986, cited in Oakley 1992: 27) is comprehensive in its coverage of most aspects of support:

> The domain assigned to social support varies from the expansive view that support is the overriding construct for the provision of social relationships, to the specifically focused view that support is information, nurturance, empathy, encouragement, validating behaviour, constructive, genuineness, sharedness and reciprocity, instrumental help, or recognition of competence. The nature and specificity of each definition of social support depends on the study for which it was designed.

Whilst Brown's (1986) definition of social support is broad, we would also add financial and spiritual support to this definition as we believe they are important components of social support. Although there are different definitions of social support, researchers agree that social support is about relationships (Oakley 1992). However, relationships are not always supportive (Oakley 1992). Individuals who receive social support feel loved and valued by others and feel connected to a larger social network (Gramling and Auerbach 2006). Thus, broadly speaking, social support has many elements – financial, informational, emotional, practical and spiritual.

Researchers have attempted to define social support. Kitamura and colleagues (1999) identify three components of received support – emotional, informational and instrumental (practical). The first component, emotional support, is defined as feeling validated and understood by others and having someone to talk to when difficulties arise. Emotional support also includes empathy, encouragement, recognition of competence and nurturance (Brown, 1986 cited in Oakley 1992). A woman's social network is important for feedback about her competence as a mother (Mercer 1981; Rubin 1984). The second aspect, informational support, refers to people who advise and guide us through difficulties (Kitamura et al. 1999) or provide information to anticipate the difficulties. The third component, instrumental or practical support, refers to someone who is competent to perform duties such as childcare and helps with household chores (Beck 1998; Kitamura et al. 1999).

There are two important aspects of social support – perceived (expected) and received (tangible) social support (Barrera 1986; Kitamura et al. 1999). Perceived support refers to the expectation of future social support by one or more people, as well as the quality of this support (Kitamura et al. 1999). Received support refers to the actual support given to individuals when they require it (Kitamura et al. 1999). Morriss and Morriss (2000: 428) suggest that received support can prevent and reduce the length of depressive episodes and is highlighted in the following quote:

> The most consistent findings linking social support to the onset or outcome of depressive episodes relate to the patient's perception that social support is present and effective.

In the literature, there are conflicting findings as to the number of people that individuals need to provide social support. Stoppard (1999) illustrated that social support is determined by the quality and quantity of social relationships and social networks. Similarly, Beck (1998) revealed the number of support members in a woman's support network, as well as the distance from support members, and the frequency of contact were important elements of social support. However, Tracey and Abell (1994) found that the number or location of support people was unrelated to the quality of social support.

3.3   Chapter Summary

This chapter has provided a broad overview of the biomedical and sociological theoretical perspectives and treatments for PND. The biopsychosocial model provides a holistic approach to health care. This chapter has explored two previous models as they acknowledge the psychosocial factors that contribute to depression and PND, such as loss and relationship difficulties. There are limitations of using only the biomedical model as it ignores the social, cultural and personal factors contributing to PND, such as gender, significant life events, cultural differences and the lack of support.

In this chapter, we have also examined the importance of social support for an individual's emotional well-being. Researchers have identified that social support is the most important variable to consider when investigating PND, as the lack of support has been linked to PND. However, there is a scant amount of literature investigating the types of support women require in the postpartum period to assist with their adjustment to motherhood.

The next chapter will examine women's childhood, pregnancy and childbirth experiences and the couples' perceptions of PND before diagnosis.

References

American Psychiatric Association. (2000). *Diagnostic and statistical manual of mental disorders, text revision. DSM-IV-TR* (4 revisedth ed.). Washington, DC: American Psychiatric Press.
Anand, A., & Charney, D. S. (2000). Norepinephrine dysfunction in depression. *Journal of Clinical Psychiatry, 61*(10), 16–24.
Appleby, L., Warner, R., Whitton, A., & Faragher, B. (1997). A controlled study of fluoxetine and cognitive-behavioural counselling in the treatment of postnatal depression. *British Medical Journal, 314*(7085), 932–936.

Austin, M. P., & Lumley, J. (2003). Antenatal screening for postnatal depression: A systematic review. *Acta Psychiatrica Scandinavia, 107*(1), 10–17.

Barrera, M. (1986). Distinctions between social support concepts, measures, and models. *American Journal of Community Psychology, 14*, 413–445.

Bebbington, P. E. (1998). Sex and depression. *Psychological Medicine, 28*(1), 1–8.

Beck, C. T. (1992). The lived experience of postpartum depression: A phenomenological study. *Nursing Research, 41*(3), 166–170.

Beck, C. T. (1993). Teetering on the edge: A substantive theory of postpartum depression. *Nursing Research, 42*, 42–48.

Beck, C. T. (1996). Postpartum depressed mothers' experiences interacting with their children. *Nursing Research, 45*, 98–104.

Beck, C. T. (1998). A checklist to identify women at risk for developing postpartum depression. *Journal of Obstetric, Gynecologic, & Neonatal Nursing, 27*(1), 39–46.

Beck, C. T. (1999). Postpartum depression: Stopping the thief that steals motherhood. *AWHONN Lifelines, 3*(4), 41–44.

Beck, C. T. (2002). Theoretical perspectives of postpartum depression and their treatment implications. *The American Journal of Maternal/Child Nursing, 27*(5), 282–287.

Berggren-Clive, K. (1998). Out of the darkness and into the light: Women's experiences with depression of childbirth. *Canadian Journal of Community Mental Health, 17*, 103–120.

Borjesson, B., Paperin, C., & Lindell, M. (2004). Maternal support during the first year of infancy. *Journal of Advanced Nursing, 45*(6), 588–594.

Borrell-Carrio, F., Suchman, A. L., & Epstein, R. M. (2004). The biopsychosocial model 25 years later: Principles, practice, and scientific inquiry. *Annals of Family Medicine, 2*(6), 576–582.

Brown, G. W. (1998). Genetic and population perspectives on life events and depression. *Social Psychiatry & Psychiatric Epidemiology, 33*, 363–372.

Brown, G. W., & Harris, T. (1978). *Social origins of depression. A study of psychiatric disorder in women.* London: Tavistock Publications Limited.

Brown, G. W., Andrews, B., & Harris, T. O. (1986). Social support, self esteem and depression. *Psychological Medicine, 16*, 813–831.

Brown, S., Lumley, J., Small, R., & Astbury, J. (1994). *Missing voices. The experience of motherhood.* Australia: Oxford University Press.

Brown, G. W., Harris, T. O., & Hepworth, C. (1995). Loss, humiliation and entrapment among women developing depression: A patient and non-patient comparison. *Psychological Medicine, 25*(1), 7–22.

Brown, M. A. (1986). Social support during pregnancy: A unidimensional or multidimensional construct? *Nursing Research, 35*(1), 4–9.

Brugha, T. S. (1995). *Social support and psychiatric disorder: Research findings and guidelines for clinical practice.* Cambridge: Cambridge University Press.

Buist, A. (2006). Perinatal depression. Assessment and management. *Australian Family Physician, 35*(9), 670–673.

Buist, A., Barnett, B., Milgrom, J., Pope, S., Condon, J. T., Ellwood, D. A., et al. (2002). To screen or not to screen- that is the question in perinatal depression. *The Medical Journal of Australia, 177*(7 October), S101–S105.

Burrows, G, & Norman, T. (2001). Depressive disorders. *MediMedia*, 1–6.

Busfield, J. (1996). *Men, women and madness. Understanding gender and mental disorder.* London: MacMillan.

Cacioppo, J. T. (1994). Social neuroscience: Autonomic, neuroendocrine, and immune responses to stress. *Psychophysiology, 31*, 113–128.

Chan, S., & Levy, V. (2004). Postnatal depression: A qualitative study of the experiences of a group of Hong-Kong Chinese women. *Journal of Clinical Nursing, 13*, 120123.

Chan, S. W. C., Levy, V., Chung, T. K. H., & Lee, D. (2002). A qualitative study of the experiences of a group of Hong Kong Chinese women diagnosed with postnatal depression. *Journal of Advanced Nursing, 39*(6), 571–579.

Cleare, A. J., Murray, R. M., & O'Keane, V. (1997). Do noradrenergic reuptake inhibitors affect serotonergic function in depression? *Psychopharmacology, 134*, 406–410.

Creedy, D., & Shochet, I. (1996). Caring for women suffering from depression in the postnatal period. *Australian and New Zealand Journal of Mental Health Nursing, 5*, 13–19.

Davar, B. (1999). *The mental Health of Indian women: A feminist agenda*. New Delhi: Sage.

Drew, S. (2003). *Stranger in the community- life after cancer in childhood*. Unpublished PhD, University of Melbourne, Melbourne.

Eaker, E. D. (2005). Social support and physical health: Understanding the health consequences of relationships. *American Journal of Epidemiology, 161*(3), 297–298.

Engel, G. L. (1977). The need for a new medical model: A challenge for biomedicine. *Science, 196*, 129–136.

Engel, G. L. (1980). The clinical application of the biopsychosocial model. *American Journal of Psychiatry, 137*(5), 535–544.

Eriksen, K., & Kress, V. E. (2005). *Beyond the DSM story*. Thousand Oaks: Sage.

Ferrer, R. L., Palmer, R., Burge, S. K. (2005). The Family Contribution to Health Status: A Population-Level Estimate. *Annals of Family Medicine* 3(2): 102–108.

Finlay-Jones, R. (1989). Anxiety. In G. W. Brown & T. O. Harris (Eds.), *Life events and illness*. New York: Guilford Press.

Fullager, S., & Gattuso, S. (2002). Rethinking gender, risk and depression in Australian mental health policy. *Australian e-Journal for the Advancement of Mental Health, 1*(3), 1–13.

Gordon, J. H., Borison, R. L., & Diamond, B. I. (1980). Modulation of dopamine receptor sensitivity by estrogen. *Biological Psychiatry, 15*, 389–396.

Gottlieb, L. N., & Mendelson, M. J. (1995). Mothers' moods and social support when a second child is born. *Maternal-Child Nursing Journal, 23*(1), 3–14.

Gramling, S. E., & Auerbach, S. (2006). *Stress (psychology) Microsoft Encarta online encyclopedia*. http://www.encarta.msn.com/text_761572052__0/Stress_(psychology).html. Accessed 23 May 2006.

Hanson, R. W. (2007). Biopsychosocial model of pain. http://www.long-beach.med.va.gov/Our_Services/Patient_Care/cpmpbook/cpmp-3.html. Accessed 28 Mar 2007.

Harbuz, M. (2002). Neuroendocrine function and chronic inflammatory stress. *Experimental Physiology, 87*(5), 519–525.

Harmer, C. J., Hill, S. A., Taylor, M. J., Cowen, P. J., & Goodwin, G. M. (2003). Toward a neuropsychological theory of antidepressant drug action: Increase in positive emotional bias after potentiation of norepinephrine activity. *American Journal of Psychiatry, 160*(5), 990–992.

Harris, T. (2001). Recent developments in understanding the psychosocial aspects of depression. *British Medical Bulletin, 57*, 17–32.

Huang, Y. C., & Mathers, N. (2001). Postnatal depression- biological or cultural? A comparative study of postnatal women in the UK and Taiwan. *Journal of Advanced Nursing, 33*(3), 279–287.

Kendler, K. S., Thornton, L. M., & Gardner, C. O. (2000). Stressful life events and previous episodes in the etiology of major depression in women: An evaluation of the "Kindling" hypothesis. *American Journal of Psychiatry, 157*, 1243–1251.

Kendler, K. S., Gardner, C. O., & Prescott, C. A. (2002). Toward a comprehensive developmental model for major depression in women. *American Journal of Psychiatry, 159*(7), 1133–1145.

Kinard, E. M. (1990). *Depression and social support in mothers of abused children*. Paper presented at the annual meeting of the American Public Health Association, New York.

Kitamura, T., Kijima, N., Watanabe, K., Takezaki, Y., & Tanaka, E. (1999). Precedents of perceived social support: Personality and early life experiences. *Psychiatry and Clinical Neurosciences, 53*, 649–654.

Kitzinger, S. (1992). *Ourselves as mothers. The universal experience of motherhood*. London: Doubleday.

Kwok, W. L. (2003). *Postnatal depression in Whittlesea*. A discussion paper, The North Central Metropolitan Primary Care Partnership.

Lawrie, T., Herxheimer, A., & Dalton, K. (2003). Oestrogens and progestogens for preventing and treating postnatal depression (Cochrane Review). In: *The Cochrane Library*, Issue 3, Oxford: Update Software.

Leonard, B. E. (2001). Stress, norepinephrine and depression. *Journal of Psychiatry and Neuroscience, 26*, S11–S16.

Mauthner, N. S. (1999). "Feeling low and feeling really bad about feeling low": Women's experiences of motherhood and postpartum depression. *Canadian Psychology, 40*(2), 143–161.

Mauthner, N. S. (2002). *The darkest days of my life. Stories of postpartum depression*. Cambridge: Harvard University Press.

Mercer, R. T. (1981). A theoretical framework for studying factors that impact on the maternal role. *Nursing Research, 30*, 73–77.

Milgrom, J., Martin, P. R., & Negri, L. M. (1999). *Treating postnatal depression. A psychological approach for health care practitioners*. Chichester: Wiley.

Morriss, K. M., & Morriss, E. E. (2000). Contextual evaluation of social adversity in the management of depressive disorder. *Advances in Psychiatric Treatment, 6*, 423–431.

Morrow, M., Smith, J., Lai, Y., & Jaswal, S. (2008). Shifting landscapes: Immigrant women and post partum depression. *Health Care for Women International, 29*(6), 593–617.

Nahas, V. L., & Amasheh, N. (1999). Culture care meanings and experiences of postpartum depression among Jordanian Australian women: A transcultural study. *Journal of Transcultural Nursing, 10*, 37–45.

Nahas, V. L., Hillege, S., & Amasheh, N. (1999). International exchange. Postpartum depression: The lived experiences of Middle Eastern migrant women in Australia. *Journal of Nurse-Midwifery, 44*(1), 65–74.

National Health and Medical Research Council. (2000). Postnatal depression. A systematic review of published scientific literature to 1999. http://www.nhmrc.gov.au/publications/synopses/wh29syn.htm. Accessed 12 June 2007.

Nazroo, J. Y., Edwards, A. C., & Brown, G. W. (1997). Gender differences in the onset of depression following a shared life event: A study of couples. *Psychological Medicine, 27*, 9–19.

Novack, D. H. (2003). Realizing Engel's vision: Psychosomatic medicine and the education of physician-healers. *Psychosomatic Medicine, 65*, 925–930.

Oakley, A. (1992). *Social support and motherhood. The natural history of a research project*. Oxford: Blackwell.

Oshimer, A., Miyano, H., Yamashita, S., Owashi, T., Suzuki, S., Sakano, Y., et al. (2001). Psychological, autonomic and neuroendocrine responses to acute stressors in the combined dexamethasone/CRH test: A study in healthy subjects. *Journal of Psychiatric Research, 35*, 95–104.

Patel, V. (2001). Cultural factors and international epidemiology. *British Medical Bulletin, 57*, 33–45.

Raeburn, J. M., & Rootman, I. (1989). Towards an expanded health field concept: Conceptual and research issues in a new era of health promotion. *Health Promotion, 3*, 383–392.

Ray, K. L, & Hodnett, E. D. (2006). Caregiver support for postpartum depression. *Cochrane Database for Systematic Reviews, 1*, No page number.

Rubin, R. (1984). *Maternal identity and the maternal experience*. New York: Springer.

Sagud, M., Hotujac, L., Peles, A. M., & Jakovljevic, M. (2002). Gender differences in depression. *Colegium Antropologicum, 26*(1), 149–157.

Seligman, M. E., & Rosenhan, D. L. (1998). *Abnormality*. New York: W.W. Norton & Company.

Smith, R., Cubis, J., Brinstead, M., Lewis, T., Singh, B., & Owens, P. (1989). Mood changes, obstetric experience and alterations in plasma cortisol, [beta]-endorphin and corticotrophin releasing hormone during pregnancy and the puerperium. *Journal of Psychosomatic Research, 34*, 53–69.

Stewart, S., & Jambunathan, J. (1996). Hmong women and postpartum depression. *Health Care for Women International, 17*, 319–330.

Stocky, A. (1992). Psychiatry's model and measurement. In J. Carter (Ed.), *Postnatal depression: Towards a research agenda for human services and health.* Canberra: Commonwealth of Australia.

Stoppard, J. M. (1999). Why new perspectives are needed for understanding depression in women. *Canadian Psychology, 40*(2), 79–90.

Tracey, E. M., & Abell, N. (1994). Social network mapping: Some future refinements on administration. *Social Work Research, 18,* 57–60.

Ugarriza, D. N. (2002). Postpartum depressed women''s explanation of depression. *Journal of Nursing Scholarship, 34*(3), 227–233.

United States Food and Drug Administration (FDA). (2005). FDA Talk Paper. T05-25. FDA reviews data for antidepressant use in adults. http://www.fda.gov/cder/drug/advisory/SSR1200507.htm. Accessed 15 July 2005.

Victorian Drug Usage Advisory Committee. (2003). *Therapeutic guidelines: Psychotropic* (5th ed.). North Melbourne: BPA Print Group.

WHO. (2000). *Women's mental health. An evidenced based review.* Geneva: WHO.

WHO. (2001). Mental health: Strengthening mental health promotion. http://www.who.int/mediacentre/factsheets/fs220/en/. Accessed 12 June 2007.

Wieck, A., Kumar, R., Hirst, A. D., Marks, M. N., Campbell, I. C., & Checkley, S. A. (1991). Increased sensitivity of dopamine receptors and recurrence of affective psychosis after childbirth. *British Medical Journal, 303,* 613–616.

Wisner, K. L., Parry, B. L., & Piontek, C. M. (2002). Postpartum depression. *The New England Journal of Medicine, 347*(3), 194–199.

Wood, A. F., Thomas, S. P., Droppleman, P. G., & Meighan, M. (1997). The downward spiral of postpartum depression. *Maternal-Child Nursing Journal, 22,* 308–317.

Chapter 4
'Kept in the Dark': Childhood, Pregnancy and Childbirth Experiences

> I just needed to be reminded what was going on. I don't like to be kept in the dark. I kept
> saying, "Is the baby alright?" because they put the probes in his head (Samantha).

Samantha's quote highlights the need for information and support in childbirth from health professionals. In this chapter, we will explore women's childhood, pregnancy and childbirth experiences. What was evident from the couples' stories was the need for support from health professionals and the importance of a female role model to learn the skills of motherhood. This chapter will detail the significant life events that the women experienced in childhood, pregnancy and childbirth that they perceive contributed to their PND. Brown and Harris (1978), while identifying pregnancy and childbirth as significant events, consider other life events which could impact on pregnancy and the amount of loss that women experienced from such events.

'Kept in the dark' represents women and their partners' experiences with health professionals in pregnancy and childbirth, and was a term used by one of the participants. Women's childhood, pregnancy and childbirth experiences will be discussed in a temporal order. This will be followed by women and their partners' perceptions of PND before diagnosis. The lack of information about PND from health professionals, combined with the sensationalisation of PND in the media, resulted in confusion about the severity of the illness.

4.1 Childhood Experiences

Most women voiced unhappy memories of their childhood, which were tarnished by the feeling of being unloved and rejected, and/or the experience of abuse. These categories created a major barrier in communication particularly between women and their own mothers. Several researchers contend that women with abusive and dysfunctional families of origin are at increased risk of developing depression (Barlow et al. 2006; Brown and Anderson 1991; Brown et al. 1996; Buist 1996,

C. Westall and P. Liamputtong, *Motherhood and Postnatal Depression: Narratives of Women and Their Partners*, DOI 10.1007/978-94-007-1694-0_4,
© Springer Science+Business Media B.V. 2011

1998; Martins and Gaffan 2000; WHO 2000). There is evidence that childhood difficulties may contribute to depression as individuals can experience long-term damage to their self-esteem or may experience difficulty attaching to others (Brown and Harris 1978; Harris 2001; WHO 2000). Boyce (2003) makes a link between the quality of parenting that women receive in childhood with their ability to cope with motherhood. Poor parenting, such as the lack of parental care, has also been associated with the later development of PND (Boyce et al. 1991).

4.1.1 Feeling Unloved and Rejected

Some women felt rejected and unloved by their own mothers when they were children, and they carried these feelings into their adult lives. As adults, they expected to be supported emotionally and to have a deeper relationship with their mothers. Women also perceived a continuing sense of rejection when their mothers were reluctant to visit them after the birth, or remained emotionally and/or physically distant. Melissa discussed how she felt rejected as a child as her mother was unable to tell her that she loved her. She had constant nightmares of her mother abandoning her:

> When I was a teenager there was a lot of angst between my mother and I, we didn't see eye to eye. I used to get very upset because I couldn't ever remember her telling me that she loved me – never, and that upset me…I used to have nightmares that my mother had disowned me, it was a recurring nightmare – she didn't like me, and she was getting rid of me.

Similarly, Kris felt unloved by her mother and blamed herself for their distant relationship. She was also haunted at night by thoughts that her mother did not love her and wanted her to grow up so she could enjoy her life:

> I blamed myself for our lack of relationship I suppose and thinking why doesn't she love me enough? Why doesn't she want to be with me?…I felt like she couldn't wait for me to get to what she considered a reasonable age so that she could go and live her life…because I think that was a big part of the problem that I would wake up at night and cry, and questioning what did I do wrong? Why doesn't she love me?

Gottlieb and Mendelson (1995) contend that feeling loved and accepted is an important component of emotional support and can improve self-esteem. Studies have shown that individuals, who perceived that they were rejected as children, were more likely to carry these feelings of rejection into their adult lives (Hurst 1999; Sluckin 1998) and to develop PND (Crockenberg and Leerkes 2003). Rubin (1967a) describes the child as an extension of self. Therefore, any rejection of the child is seen as a rejection of the women themselves.

Some women in our study also experienced abuse in their childhoods that in some cases created a barrier to communication between women and their own mothers.

4.1.2 Abuse (The Hidden Barrier to Communication)

The majority of women disclosed a history of childhood sexual abuse, and one woman disclosed a history of adult rape. Most of the episodes of sexual abuse that women experienced involved penetration; the perpetrators were fathers, brothers and uncles, and occurred over months or years. In the literature, incestuous abuse is more likely to occur more than once, and over a longer period of time, compared with non-incestuous abuse (Fleming 1997).

Sexual abuse of a child is an act of power where the child is involved in sexual activity, and the child has not been protected by the child's parent or caregiver (Department of Human Services 2007). Girls are twice as likely to be sexually abused compared with boys (Critchley 1996; Harris 2001). Despite the frequency of sexual abuse amongst girls, most studies investigating PND have failed to ask about past sexual abuse. In Australia, Critchley (1996) estimated that 20–25% of girls and 15% of boys are victims of child sexual abuse. Harris (2001) proposed that gender differences in rates of depression could perhaps be explained by the higher rates of sexual abuse in girls. The higher incidence of child sexual abuse for women participants is consistent with Palmer, Coleman, Chaloner, Oppenheimer and Smith's findings (1993) that women with a psychiatric disorder are two to three times more likely to have experienced childhood sexual abuse. In our study, the high disclosure of sexual abuse could be due to the fact that in-depth interviews were conducted, and the established rapport and sensitivity provided during the process of interviewing. One participant who attended Carolyn's postnatal support group commented that she would have been unable to disclose her abusive past if she had not known her previously. Despite this comment, women whom we had no previous contact with were very open talking about their experiences of past abuse.

Sexual abuse can damage a child physically, emotionally and behaviourally (Department of Human Services 2007), and can result in feelings of personal shame, betrayal, and powerlessness (Westall 2001). If the abused child is not believed, the abuse is likely to continue and result in long-term damage (Department of Human Services 2007). Our participants, even years after the abuse, were unable to tell others what had happened to them, particularly their partners and mothers. This finding is supported by evidence that sexual abuse is a secret that may be carried for years by abused individuals, resulting in feelings of isolation and disconnection from others (Westall 2001).

Even at the time of interview, one woman was unable to tell her husband that she had been sexually abused as a child. Another woman, who was sexually abused, was in a domestic violence situation with her husband. Another woman was raped as an adult. In the literature, there is evidence that women who have experienced sexual abuse are also vulnerable to further abuse and exploitation (Department of Human Services 2007), and are more likely to be raped as adults or in relationships where there is domestic violence (Mullen and Fleming 1998; Smith 1998a, b; Tilley 2000). David, whose wife Kim was raped as an adult, discussed the 'barrier' between his wife and her mother when she was unable to tell her mother about her experience of adult rape. This partner disclosed his wife's experience of rape during the focus group:

> When she was about eighteen she was raped…and she's never, ever told her mum that that happened… There's always been a barrier between her and her mother.

Women also carried the secret of their past sexual abuse into their adult lives. These women discussed their expectation as children that their mothers would stop the abuse and do something about it. They discussed their disappointment with their own mothers when they failed to protect them from abuse, especially when some of the mothers were also sexually abused. The Department of Human Services (2007) reported that the most serious effects of past abuse occur as a result of no-one stopping the abuse or protecting the child. In our study, the anger and resentment these women experienced continued to haunt them in their adult lives. Kath was 'angry' that her mother, who was also sexually abused, was unable to stop the abuse and keep her safe. She remarked:

> And she [mother] tells me a cousin did the same thing [sexual abuse] to her, so then it makes me angry. Why didn't she protect me?

Melissa also wanted her mother to protect her from the sexual abuse. As an adult, she discussed feeling 'resentment' towards her mother for not being aware of the ongoing abuse and stopping it:

> When I became a teenager I think I harboured a lot of resentment towards my mother for not knowing something was wrong [sexual abuse] and doing something about it.

Several women, who were abused in childhood, discussed being depressed in their teenage years and early twenties as a result of their past sexual abuse. Women who were sexually abused as children claimed they felt isolated and different to others as a result of their past abuse. These women reported how their past abuse resulted in the loss of self-esteem and self-worth. As a teenager, Danni blamed herself for leading the perpetrator on. It took years for her to accept that the perpetrator was wrong. She discussed the long-term damage to her self-esteem and self-respect as a result of her past abuse:

> I think it [child sexual abuse] does a lot of damage to your self-esteem and your self-respect. I think a lot of women who have been sexually abused feel like they deserve it somehow. I used to wonder when I was a teenager what I did to lead him [perpetrator] on but now that I'm an adult that was a really warped way of thinking. It wasn't my fault. But on top of me grieving for my mum and getting depressed about her dying, then being sexually abused on top of that I reckon that would have been a huge contributing factor to my underlying depression anyway.

The women commonly reported problems with intimacy in their relationships with their partners. Researchers have argued that relationship problems are common when women have experienced past sexual abuse (Department of Human Services 2007; Hennebry 1998). Kath discussed the problems with intimacy as a result of her past sexual abuse. In her marital relationship, the past abuse created a wedge in their relationship as she misinterpreted her husband's need for affection:

> He gets obsessed about sex… He thought because I didn't want sex I didn't love him, and it was sort of a vicious circle. He tries to be very supportive but I misread some things that he does. [He] tries to be affectionate and I see it as sexual.

In the literature, there is evidence that adult survivors of sexual abuse are more likely to develop depression than non-abused women (Buist 1998; Finkelhor 1984; Hegarty et al. 2004; Mullen and Fleming 1998; Pearson 1993; Raphael-Leff 2000; Rhodes and Hutchinson 1994; Smith 1998a, b; Tilley 2000; WHO 2000). The long-term effects of child sexual abuse can be devastating as it can affect not only a woman's sexuality but also her sexual identity, self-image and self-esteem (Pearson 1993; Raphael-Leff 2000; Rhodes and Hutchinson 1994; Tilley 2000). Women who have experienced sexual abuse are at risk of self-abuse, prostitution, poor parenting, suicide attempts or post-traumatic stress disorder (Buist 1997; Elders and Albert 1998; Hennebry 1998). These women may also have drug and alcohol problems, and eating disorders (Bachman et al. 1988; Mullen and Fleming 1998; Smith 1998a, b).

The safety of children in the family environment is a shared responsibility between the family, the community and the government (Department of Human Services 2007). In Victoria, health professionals are mandated to report cases of suspected child sexual abuse to the Child Protection Service. The abused child is offered counselling and support to reduce self-blame and the detrimental long-term effects of the abuse (Department of Human Services 2007).

In summary, some women carried the secret of sexual abuse through pregnancy and childbirth because it was never discussed, or raised, or they choose not to disclose such a history (Westall 2001). However, health professionals can sensitively ask women about a history of sexual abuse when women are asked about their past medical, surgical and obstetrical histories. Pregnancy is an opportune time to ask women about a history of childhood sexual abuse and to determine the need for counselling.

4.2   Pregnancy Experiences

Pregnancy is not only a biological event but also an adaptive process (Brockington 1996), and is a critical time for the development of mood disorders (Ross et al. 2005). Most women in our study had planned pregnancies. However, they expressed the need for support during pregnancy when they experienced anxiety related to unresolved grief from previous perinatal losses (miscarriages, foetal death in utero, terminations and adoption) and abnormal results from antenatal testing. The importance of support in pregnancy has been documented in the literature. Researchers have found that support provided during pregnancy can improve maternal and foetal well-being and can even increase the weight of the baby at birth (Oakley 1992). Women with inadequate social support in pregnancy are more likely to report poorer health, book later prenatal care, seek medical help more frequently and be depressed after the birth (Webster et al. 2000).

4.2.1   Anxiety from Past Perinatal Losses

A large number of women in our study experienced perinatal losses – ten women experienced at least one miscarriage (ranges from one to three miscarriages), one woman terminated her pregnancy due to a foetal congenital anomaly (anencephaly), one woman experienced a foetal death in utero and another woman experienced a form of perinatal loss when she put her baby up for adoption. In Australia, a miscarriage is defined as pregnancy loss occurring before 20 weeks gestation (Sydney 2007). The incidence of perinatal losses for women participants is equivalent to the rough estimate that 20% or more of all pregnancies result in pregnancy loss (Cote-Arsenault and Mahlangu 1999). Perinatal losses are becoming more prevalent due to assisted reproduction, such as in vitro fertilisation (IVF) and antenatal testing (Bennett et al. 2005).

Women, who experienced perinatal losses, were anxious during their pregnancies and feared they would lose the subsequent pregnancy. These findings have been reported in other studies (see Cote-Arsenault and Mahlangu 1999; Thuet et al. 1988). There is evidence that anxiety is a precursor to PND (American Psychiatric Association 2000; Austin 2003; Buist 2002; Matthey et al. 2003; O'Connor et al. 2002; Ross et al. 2003). Matthey and colleagues (2003) claimed that anxiety may be more of a predictor for PND than a history of depression, and concluded that anxiety and depression need to be assessed in pregnancy.

The source of women's anxieties, when women later develop PND, has not been explored in sufficient depth in the literature. Cote-Arsenault (2003) studied 160 women and found that women who experienced perinatal losses were more anxious with their subsequent pregnancies. Women with a history of perinatal loss were more concerned about their pregnancies and babies compared with women without a history of perinatal loss. Cote-Arsenault (2003) argued that women's heightened anxiety needs to be acknowledged and more frequent visits with the health professional must be arranged.

In our study, the feeling of anxiety robbed women of the opportunity of enjoying their pregnancy experiences. Maria was anxious during her second pregnancy following a miscarriage. She also described emotionally detaching herself from the pregnancy. Maria and Kyle were both 'surprised' when they were discharged from the hospital with a live baby, as Maria commented:

> [I was] very anxious and concerned about how and what would happen [with the next pregnancy].... We [Kyle and I] had, without thinking about it, got prepared for [the fact] that she wouldn't even be alive when she was born, so we were a bit surprised when we were bringing a baby home.

The impact of miscarriage on emotional well-being has been well documented. Researchers have argued that women who experience perinatal losses are more likely to develop PND (Milgrom et al. 1999). Also, researchers have found a link between pregnancy loss and unresolved grief and anxiety (Brockington 1996; Cote-Arsenault and Mahlangu 1999). Some researchers claim that 15–20% of women who experience perinatal loss have significant adjustment problems with the next pregnancy, and many seek professional help (Hughes et al. 2002; Klier et al. 2000; Swanson 1999). Increased rates of mental health problems following perinatal losses have also been reported (Fox 2007; Hughes et al. 2002; Vance et al. 1995). Hughes and associates (2002) found that approximately 20% of women who experienced perinatal loss developed prolonged depression and a further 20% developed post-traumatic stress disorder (PTSD).

In our study, it was women's reaction to their perinatal losses that affected their emotional well-being following the loss, not the gestational age of the foetus at the time of the loss. Similarly, Cote-Arsenault and Mahlangu (1999) found that the attachment to the pregnancy was unrelated to the gestational age of the baby and was different for all women. Even reassuring kicks from the baby and ultrasounds showing the foetal heart beating were not enough to reassure women participants who had experienced perinatal losses that their babies would be born alive. However, our findings differed from that of Cote-Arsenault and Mahlangu (1999) which say that women's anxieties were not reduced after they had reached the gestation of their previous loss (or milestones), rather their anxiety continued right through their pregnancies and even after the birth. This difference in findings could be an important factor in the later development of PND. Maria discussed the impact of her miscarriage on her emotional well-being when she stated, 'I couldn't see how I could ever get better after such a great loss'. Katie experienced a miscarriage with her first pregnancy. She had difficulty enjoying her second pregnancy in case she lost the baby again:

> When I actually did fall pregnant with the next child it was a pretty [pause] stressful time because in a way I wasn't allowing myself to feel the joy of a new pregnancy in case something went wrong.

Most women received no counselling for their perinatal losses and were given little opportunity to grieve. Mary discussed the lack of counselling she received following two miscarriages:

> There were two of those [miscarriages]… there was no counselling or anything. It was just like, "It's happened get on with your life".

Losing a baby is the loss of a life and the loss of a dream of becoming a mother or father. The bereavement literature has focused on the death of a loved one rather than pregnancy losses (Tsartsara and Johnson 2006). In congruence with the findings from our study, Cote-Arsenault (1995, 2003, 2004) argued that women had lost babies, not pregnancies. For women, the impact of perinatal loss may continue years after the loss (Cote-Arsenault and Mahlangu 1999). Researchers have found that women experience traumatic grief as a result of perinatal loss (Pasternak et al. 1991; Prigerson et al. 1999). Health professionals advocate for the resolution of grief before contemplating another pregnancy (Cuisinier et al. 1996). Pasternak and others (1991) argued that traumatic grief is a separate category to depression and needs further investigation. The unresolved grief that women in our study experienced had a profound impact on their subsequent pregnancies and their attachment to their babies before and after the birth. Health professionals play a crucial role in identifying the need for counselling for women who experience perinatal losses.

4.2.2   Emotional Detachment from the Pregnancy

Several women, who experienced perinatal losses, detached themselves from subsequent pregnancies as they feared they would lose their babies. Similar findings have been reported by other researchers (see Cote-Arsenault and Mahlangu 1999; Hense 1994; Thuet et al. 1988). Despite the advances in technology, there is limited research on the impact of perinatal losses on subsequent pregnancies. Our study reflects the findings of Cote-Arsenault and Mahlangu (1999), namely the women were unable to enjoy subsequent pregnancies, had received no counselling for their perinatal losses and were expected to continue their lives as if their losses had never occurred. Normally during pregnancy, ultrasounds and foetal movement are reassuring to women (Brockington 1996). In contrast, our participants who had previously experienced pregnancy losses were not reassured by ultrasounds and kicks from the baby, and as a result, they often remained detached from their babies until after the birth. Ursula discussed how she remained 'detached' throughout her second pregnancy as she feared she would lose her baby:

> I think you go along, you don't want to get too attached in case it [miscarriage] happens again, and I remember saying that even if you get to thirty weeks you're still not safe because things can happen…Until that baby's in your arms you don't know that everything's okay. I think that's sort of how I was right through the pregnancy – a bit detached.

Women perceived that the disconnection with their foetuses in pregnancy resulted in delayed bonding with their babies after the birth. This delay in bonding started either straight after the birth or when women were discharged from hospital.

Brockington (1996) argues that the strength of the maternal bond in pregnancy influences the mother-infant attachment after the birth. Beatrice, however, distanced herself from her second pregnancy to protect herself from getting attached to a baby that may not survive. When she was pregnant following a miscarriage, she described her pregnancy as a 'medical dilemma'. Despite a reassuring ultrasound at 5 months gestation, Beatrice remained anxious and detached herself from her baby before the birth. She discussed the bonding difficulties after the birth occurring as a result of her anxiety during the pregnancy:

> The first one [pregnancy], I think my way of coping with it was to treat the whole thing as a medical dilemma and distance the whole thing from actually producing a live baby… It wasn't until the ultrasound around 5 months–20 weeks, when I could see him and he was moving, that I allowed myself to think, "I'm having a baby". No doubt that's got something to do with how I reacted afterwards. That act of separation during the pregnancy came back after he was born and I had trouble bonding with him.

Although Tessa did not experience a perinatal loss, she felt emotionally detached from her first pregnancy. When she found out she was pregnant as planned, she described receiving the news as a 'shock' and had difficulty accepting the pregnancy. Despite being physically well during her first pregnancy, Tessa was unable to prepare for the baby until she was 7 months pregnant. She reflected back on her emotional detachment with her baby before and after the birth:

> Even though the first pregnancy was relatively planned, as planned as we were going to be able to be, it was still a shock, and emotionally I don't think I was coping too well. I loved having bumps and feeling really womanly. I really enjoyed the pregnancy. I felt I looked good so the pregnancy was positive physically. Emotionally – I didn't go down a baby aisle until I was seven months pregnant, my mum did all the baby shopping, [and] that could

have been a bit of a clue in hindsight that I hadn't fully accepted it... [After the birth] I didn't love him unconditionally when I held him. I loved him but not deeply.

Unlike other participants, Sue had the unique experience of adopting her baby out due to marital difficulties and the lack of support from her partner. She explained how she remained detached from her baby for 8 months and wanted to stay pregnant forever so she would keep the baby:

> It wasn't my child and that was the mindset that I had. It was really hard that last month though because I had stayed detached until I was eight months and I was like okay I'm in my last month I don't want to let go, I don't want to deliver, I just want to stay pregnant forever because then I get to keep him.

Later in the interview, Sue discussed her postnatal experience several years later when she had her first viable child after experiencing three losses: two associated with pregnancy (miscarriage and foetal death in utero) and one after the birth (adoption):

> I remember feeling really weird about the fact that here I had lost [other children]... and still in awe that she is mine, I'm going to keep her. I was paranoid she was going to die in her crib... All I knew was loss; loss was associated with children.

Researchers have found that the attachment to the baby begins months before the birth. Peppers and Knapp (1980) claimed that nine events contribute to the mother-child bond in pregnancy: planning the pregnancy, confirming the pregnancy, accepting the pregnancy, feeling the foetal movement, accepting the foetus as an individual, giving birth, seeing the baby, touching the baby and caring for the baby. In their study, the meaning of the pregnancy was different for everyone and was affected by assisted reproduction (such as in vitro fertilisation), preparation for the birth, the number of living children, the couple's relationship and expectations from others about having a child. Researchers have also found that one of the mother's tasks in pregnancy is 'binding in' with her baby (Cranley 1981; Rubin 1984). This process is unconscious where the women gradually recognise the foetus as separate from themselves (Cote-Arsenault and Mahlangu 1999). Along a similar vein, Mercer (1981) argued that engaging with the pregnancy is an important part of the transition to motherhood.

4.2.3   Abnormal Antenatal Testing

Several participants experienced abnormal results from blood tests and/or ultrasounds when they were pregnant, and they experienced anxiety as they were faced with the possibility of terminating their pregnancy, having a baby with Down Syndrome or giving birth to a dead baby. Women tried to cope with their abnormal tests as best they could as they painfully waited for the results of further testing. One baby out of every 40 is born with a congenital anomaly (WHO 1993). Katz-Rothman (1986) uses the term 'tentative pregnancy' to describe women's fears associated with medical procedures performed in pregnancy, such as ultrasounds and amniocentesis.

Georgia, with an unplanned second pregnancy, was told 2 weeks before her due date that her baby would be born dead. She was referred to a genetic counsellor to come to terms with the fact that her baby would not survive the birth as it was too late to terminate the pregnancy. Georgia was then told that the ultrasound was wrong. She explained the fear she faced late in pregnancy when she received the news about the abnormal ultrasound result:

> I also got told that – it was roughly around eight months – that there was something wrong with the baby, and that took two weeks of you know having to go for genetic counselling, and everything like that…They told me that he had ventriculamegaly, which is like instead of the ventricles in the brain being 3 mm, they were 33 mm. So they were basically giving me counselling saying, "He's going to be born dead"… And then it turned out that it was a mistake… And they finally turned around and said, "There's nothing wrong with your baby".

Beatrice also had an abnormal ultrasound in pregnancy and was told that there was a possibility of her baby having Down Syndrome. She chose to have an amniocentesis to determine if the baby had the condition and tried to find out as much as she could about Down Syndrome so that she could make an informed decision as to whether or not she should terminate the pregnancy:

> They [health professionals] discovered that she had a cyst on the brain which could have been linked with Down Syndrome. Especially, with time ticking on I wanted to know [the possibility of Downs]. I don't know what I would have done, but part of me thought the main thing is to have the information, and if we're having a baby with Down Syndrome, I will find out all I can about it and get myself prepared, possibly terminate, although deep down I really didn't think I would be able to do it. The amniocentesis was probably the most terrifying moment of my life; I've never felt so scared. I didn't feel like I could breathe, I could feel my stomach rising and falling up and down along the needle and I was so terrified. It's the most hideous feeling, you're not meant to have a great bloody needle in through your belly.

Along a similar vein, Katie had an abnormal blood test result (maternal serum screen or triple test) in the mid-trimester of her pregnancy. She also had a previous miscarriage. Katie discussed the increased stress when she received an abnormal test result during her pregnancy:

> Just something else to add to the stresses [of pregnancy] was I was encouraged to have the triple test, and anyway the results of that came back putting me in the higher category [at-risk]… We underwent an amniocentesis and… and the results came back… everything was okay.

There is insufficient literature investigating the communication to parents when a foetal problem is suspected (WHO 1993). Zecca et al. (2006) evaluated 82 consultations with health professionals before and after antenatal testing using amniocentesis and level II ultrasounds. They found that regardless of the severity of the anomaly (minor or serious), health professionals used a disease-centred model to communicate to their patients. Furthermore, the patients' emotional and psychosocial issues were scarcely addressed by health professionals and were addressed less frequently in the group with severe anomalies (Zecca et al. 2006).

4.3   Childbirth Experiences

Childbirth is not just a physical event, it is a significant event that changes women's lives forever and affects their physical, emotional, social and spiritual well-being (Liamputtong 2007). Giving birth changes many areas of women's lives, such as their perceptions of themselves – their self-concept and social role, and their relationships with others (Cox 1988; Seguin et al. 1995). Giving birth can be an empowering experience for some women but not for most women in our study. Two key elements that influenced women's satisfaction with their birth experiences were expectations of support from health professionals and the feeling of personal control. These factors contributed to women's emotional well-being after the birth and their feeling of competence as mothers. Similar to the findings from our study, Huack et al. (2007) found that dissatisfaction with the birth experience was due to unmet expectations of support.

Researchers have argued that inadequate support during labour can affect women's emotional well-being after the birth (Beck 2004; Czarnocka and Slade 2000; Kirkham 1983; Odent 1984; Oakley 1980; Wijma et al. 1997). In a systematic review of the literature, Hodnett et al. (2003) evaluated 15 trials involving 12,791 women to compare continuous, one-to-one intrapartum support with usual care. They found that women who received continuous intrapartum support were less likely to require analgesia, operative birth or to report dissatisfaction with their childbirth experiences. There is also evidence that receiving support in labour can reduce the length of women's labour, reduce breastfeeding problems and reduce PND (Enkin et al. 2000).

4.3.1   Traumatic Births

Most women perceived their childbirths as traumatic and used the following words when they discussed their labour and birth experiences: 'very painful', 'shocking', 'felt like a failure', 'frightened', 'out of control', 'sheer hell', 'nightmare', 'horrendous' and 'a shock'. Men used similar words to describe their partner's birth experience. Kath described her childbirth experience as 'horrible, painful, and I never want to do it again. It finished me'. Another mother, Tara, expressed the trauma and fear that she experienced in childbirth:

> I ended up having a forceps delivery and that was very traumatic – very traumatic for Ethan [partner] because he could actually see what was happening, and see the faces of the staff. He said the faces – they actually looked quite worried. They attached the forceps and were pulling and pulling, and nothing happened… When Ethan talked about it afterwards he said he just thought there wasn't going to be a baby there in the end after all of that. He was horrified by the whole thing.

Women's perceptions of their childbirth experiences as traumatic were not confined to their first childbirth experiences or to the type of delivery as the majority of women had normal vaginal deliveries. The number of women who had caesarean births in our study was less than the 30% of Australian women who had caesarean births in Australia (Australian Institute of Health and Welfare 2007).

In our study, it was women's overall satisfaction with their childbirth experience, rather than intervention in childbirth, that influenced their opinion of whether or not their births were traumatic. Overall, women expected to have adequate pain relief and to receive informational and emotional support from health professionals. Several studies support these findings (Boyce 2003; Brown et al. 1994; Goodman et al. 2004; Soet et al. 2003; Waldenstrom et al. 2004). Boyce (2003) found that regardless of the type of delivery, trauma was associated with inadequate pain relief, loss of control and a lack of information contributing to feelings of powerlessness.

Monica's traumatic birth experience was unrelated to the caesarean delivery but to the inadequate pain relief she received during the procedure. The epidural was not relieving the pain. Despite her screaming when they started cutting her abdomen, no one listened to her, and she felt helpless in the hands of the health professionals. Having no one that she knew and trusted in the operating theatre added to her feelings of vulnerability. She described her traumatic experience:

> His birth was horrific, and there is no other way to describe it… I ended up being in labour for eighteen hours, and it didn't progress so they did an emergency caesar. The epidural failed and I was aware of everything…He [partner] has walked into a room with me just screaming – blood-curdling screams because I can feel them cutting me open…There were five men in the room all telling me, "It's okay, it's normal"… No-one's responding and I'm screaming as hard as I can, and as loud as I can. I'm being as clear as I can about what the problem is, and everyone's just focusing on getting the baby out… I was upset because there was no-one there that I knew and trusted to help me. I felt really vulnerable.

As a result of Monica's traumatic birth experience, she was diagnosed with posttraumatic stress disorder 3 days after the birth. Researchers have linked traumatic births with the later development of post-traumatic stress disorder (PTSD) (Beck 2004; Creedy et al. 2000; Czarnocka and Slade 2000; Wijma et al. 1997). When Monica was asked what the triggers were for her depression, she replied:

> It absolutely had to be the birth experience for me. I don't think there's any doubt in that… It was a negative experience for me from start to finish. There wasn't anything for me to celebrate… which sounds terrible, because at the end of the day I've got a beautiful, healthy little boy but there was nothing positive for me in all of it… Now he is wonderful, and now I enjoy it but at the time I was just thinking I'd made the biggest mistake of my life… Every time I closed my eyes I relived [the birth]. That's why I think, apart from having a child who never slept [laughs], when I did get the chance to lie down all I was having was nightmares, so I was terrified. It just built itself into a cycle that I couldn't break basically.

Monica's partner Luke described her birth as 'horrific' and the sense of failure that she experienced at home and in the hospital:

> Monica was dissatisfied – she was in pain she had a traumatic caesarean. In fact I think that's probably is what kicked it [PND] all off – it was perceived pretty much as a failed sort of birth, and the fact that she felt so much pain… it was horrible. I was in the theatre with her, and she had an epidural, and I walked in and they were starting to make the incision,

and Monica was just screaming, she could feel everything. And then they started asking me, "well, what do you want to do? Can we give her a general anaesthetic?" And I said, "yes".

Unlike Monica's experience, Danni's trauma started after a normal birth in the birth centre when she needed an epidural to remove her retained placenta. After the birth, the baby was taken away and she was taken to the theatre to remove the placenta. She described this experience as traumatic and considered that it contributed to PND and affected her decision to have more children:

> After [the] delivery was shocking. I had a natural birth with him [baby], and they gave me the injection to deliver the placenta; they put Jack on to suckle, and I couldn't deliver the placenta. They [midwives] ripped him off me; I ended up downstairs for five [emphasised] hours off my head on gas. I remember being absolutely hysterically crying saying, "all I want is my son". And they went in manually and removed the placenta and it came out piece by piece. I had an epidural. I was up in stirrups and I had everything after the birth that I'd avoided during the birth. So I had a natural birth and then had major intervention after it... I had made up my mind there is no way in hell I'm ever [emphasised] having another baby. There's no way I would have had another child. What I went through after the birth with the placenta and everything else and the epidural, what happened then traumatised me for a long, long, long time... All of that was a huge contributing factor to my postnatal depression.

Nicky's trauma was related to the fear that her baby would not survive the birth and the physical pain after delivery. She also described the fear she experienced when the baby's heart rate dropped dramatically during labour:

> That was a really traumatic birth... I remember feeling very frightened because the doctors themselves seemed concerned. We only had an intern in the hospital at that time, and he didn't quite know what to do, and I was worried because [my baby's] heart rate had dropped down by half. I was worried whether he would survive the birth or not... [After the birth] I had a very big episiotomy so there was a lot of pain and discomfort afterwards.

Melissa also experienced physical pain after the birth following a traumatic birth. She felt more pain after the birth when her episiotomy became infected than during her labour:

> [My labour] was a nightmare. [It was] thirty-three hours from start to finish – intense pain all that time, it wasn't a gradual thing, it was a horrible one. I ended up having an epidural after twenty-two hours of excruciating pain. I finally got an epidural, and that was topped up about three times. Eventually [he was] forceps delivered, because the suction didn't even work, and I tore from here to eternity... I had a lot, lot of stitches, no idea how many because they gave up counting. They actually gaped and became infected, and I couldn't sit for six weeks, and that pain remains with me more than the actual thirty-three hours of labour.

Kristina was so numb from her delivery experience that she was unable to remember seeing or holding her baby after the birth. Her trauma was related to a long and painful labour that ended in a forceps delivery:

> [The birth with my son] was horrendous. It was twenty-five hours [of] sheer hell. Finally they got the epidural in, and by the time I was ready to deliver I pushed for about half an hour and I ran out of energy, I had nothing left. I just gave up, and then it was a forceps delivery... I can't remember a single thing about it – I can't remember getting him, I can't remember seeing him, I couldn't remember anything by that stage. It was really bad.

Kristina's partner, William, discussed her fear of having another epidural after her first child and how it delayed future childbearing:

> Kristina went through a very, very long labour and some issues during the labour – with them putting epidurals in… She's not a great needle person… and that frightened her a lot. I don't think it was the postnatal depression for the gap between them. I think it was more to do with having to go through that [labour] again. She was really, really worried about the epidural – even when we went into birth with Chelsea, and it took her a lot to actually say, "okay, I've got to have it [epidural] again".

Kath was a survivor of childhood sexual abuse. Her trauma was related to the intervention she received with her first delivery and the feeling of recalling the sexual abuse. Kath discussed her traumatic birth experience as a 'violation':

> I felt like I was so violated… I'd describe part of the delivery as a violation I suppose. It was so traumatic. I think because it was such a rough delivery with [my first baby]. It's just the violation came back again…because it was a lot more hands on [than the second birth].

Michael, in the focus group, discussed the trauma associated with his partner, Tessa's childbirth:

> Tessa was quite traumatised leading up to the second birth. It was a real stress for her because of the trauma of the first [birth].

Although post-traumatic stress disorder and PND are separate categories in the DSM-IV-TR, they can coexist (Birth Trauma Association 2007). Early symptoms of trauma include a dazed appearance, withdrawal or temporary amnesia (Church and Scanlan 2002). Later symptoms of PTSD include irritability, anger or intense psychological distress, followed by feelings of helplessness and panic (Rhodes and Hitchinson 1994; Tilley 2000). In the literature, there is evidence that women who have survived childhood sexual abuse can relive the trauma of their abuse in childbirth (Holz 1994; Tilley 2000; Waymire 1997; Westall 2001). Women can relive their trauma through flashbacks which are memories of the original feeling of the abuse: the smells, sounds, pain and terror (Holz 1994). Smith (1998a, b) claimed that 22% of women, who were sexually abused in childhood, suffered from post-traumatic stress disorder.

The connection between traumatic births and the later development of depression has been well researched (Brown et al. 1994; Chalmers 2002; Gamble and Creedy 2004; Gamble et al. 2005; Goodman et al. 2004; Koo et al. 2003; Oakley 1980; Odent 1984; Ryding et al. 2003; Soet et al. 2003; Selkirk et al. 2006; Waldenstrom et al. 2004; Westall 2001). Only two qualitative studies were located that explored women's experiences of birth trauma (Allen 1998; Beck 2004). Allen (1998) interviewed 20 women in the United Kingdom and found that women perceived their childbirths as traumatic if they felt they had little control, feared the baby would be harmed or had inadequate pain relief in their labours. Beck (2004) interviewed 40 women through the Internet (New Zealand, United States, Australia and United Kingdom) and found that women perceived their births as traumatic when: they had emergency caesarean deliveries; long, painful labours with inadequate pain relief; forceps deliveries; foetal or newborn deaths; premature infants and infants in the neonatal intensive care unit (NICU); degrading experiences; and perceptions of unsafe care during childbirth. Huack et al. (2007) found that a small number of participants, who expected the birth to be painful and scary, carried this fear to their next birth experience. None of the women in our study delivered prematurely. However, the lack of support affected all aspects of their care and impacted on their physical and emotional well-being, and contributed to the loss of control.

4.3.2   Loss of Control

Women's perceived loss of personal control during childbirth was an important factor in their overall satisfaction with their birth experience and was linked to women's perceptions of their births as traumatic. The loss of control was unrelated to the medicalisation of labour but to the absence of health professionals, feelings of powerlessness and lack of information about procedures and progress of labour. Past sexual abuse also contributed to the loss of control and feelings of powerlessness. Tessa experienced the loss of control in labour. The loss of control was an important issue for her in the past, and this could have been related to past abuse. She described how the loss of control she experienced in her labour may have contributed to PND:

> I lost control, and for me control had been a really important factor in the past and I think that could have contributed to the postnatal depression because I totally lost control and had a really difficult first birth.

The loss of control in childbirth has been reported in the literature (Allen 1998; Beck 2004; Czarnocka and Slade 2000; Goodman et al. 2004; Huack et al. 2007; Soet et al. 2003) and has been linked to women's negative perceptions of their childbirth experiences (Huack et al. 2007; Mackey 1995, 1998; Simkin 1991). In her research, Oakley (1980) found that women with a low level of control in labour and women who were dissatisfied with the 'management' of their labours are at risk of PND. The loss of control was not linked to the sense of failure.

However, several women in our study wanted the health professionals to take control when their labour was longer and more painful than expected. Samantha was disappointed when her second labour was longer than expected. She expected the midwife to take control for her during her second labour by giving her information about the progress of labour and the reason why the baby had to have an electrode to monitor the foetal heart rate:

> Everyone had promised me... [that my] second baby [would be] half the time, easy as that! It was exactly the opposite it was double and a half the time... My problem was [with] the first midwife, she didn't give me the reassurance and the confidence. Even though I'd done it before I'd ask her a question and I wanted to be told, I didn't want a whole range of options. [She said] "It's up to you, you can do this or do this or do this". I was almost saying everything bar just tell me what to do, I'm asking you a question "should I stand up or sit down?" and you're just saying "well it's up to you". I need you to say "sit down, Samantha". I needed someone else in control... I just needed to be reminded what was going on.

Women wanted the midwives to care for them with sensitivity and respect, and to inform them of the progress of their labours. Being present in the delivery room was also an important element of support that women needed. Kristina was 'angry' when the midwives neglected to take control for her during her first labour. She felt abandoned as none of the midwives were informing her of the progress of labour. After 15 hours of pain, the nurses informed her that she was only two centimetres dilated and was disappointed when she was not given a syntocinon infusion to augment her labour. She discussed her experience:

> I was angry that none of those nurses [midwives] took control for me at the time, and no-one said, "Okay, let's do this, let's do that", even my husband, all of them, I just thought someone should have stepped in, and I don't know done something…There should have been intervention there, they pretty much left me. I wasn't dilating, I didn't realise. I'd gone through about fifteen hours [of labour], and finally somebody decided to check how dilated I was, and I was about two centimetres, and that's when I lost it. To think I'd gone through all that for two centimetres. I thought why hadn't we known this earlier? Why hasn't someone got the syntocinon up to get me dilating?

4.3.3 Sense of Failure

A small number of women perceived they had failed when they were unable to give birth vaginally. These women received little information about caesarean sections before they delivered their babies. This lack of information from health professionals contributed to the sense of failure they experienced after the birth. Kelly discussed the sense of failure she experienced after her second caesarean delivery when she had an emergency caesarean delivery for foetal distress. In a chilling account of her birth experience, she discussed how she wanted the health professionals to leave her caesarean incision open so she could 'bleed to death':

> I just remember after when I had him I said, "you should have left the cut open so I could bleed to death". I remember saying that. I said, "I mean it because I failed again". I truly felt such a failure… The simple thing about giving birth I just couldn't even do that… I just thought what a freak.

Monica's husband, Luke, discussed his wife's expectation of having a normal delivery. When she had an emergency caesarean delivery as previously discussed, she perceived herself as a failure:

> I'm fairly sure that there was a certain expectation in Monica's mind that a natural birth was a success and anything else was a failure.

William discussed the expectation from health professionals that women will have a normal delivery and be able to breastfeed. He discussed how his wife felt like she was a failure when she had breastfeeding difficulties:

> [Health professionals] make it this rosy, beautiful picture that ninety-nine percent of people will be able to give birth naturally… [and] ninety-nine percent of people will be able to breastfeed naturally. That's another point – not everyone can breastfeed, and in some

hospitals it's rammed down your throat, "you've got to breastfeed, got to breastfeed". And even Kristina with Alex – he didn't breastfeed and attach properly... so she felt like she was failing because she couldn't breastfeed properly.

Kris too felt some failure regarding her attempt to breastfeed her baby. She remarked:

> He wasn't attaching very well. They all lose weight initially, but he probably lost more than he should. Then we came out [of hospital] he continued to lose weight. We saw the doctor and they were still pushing for me to try [to breastfeed], and it was actually Dan [partner who] got quite angry one night and just said, "go down and get bottles, this is crazy". I think that my saving in all of that was that if I hadn't breastfed my first child I would have felt quite a sense of failure and it could have been quite detrimental I think to myself.

The sense of failure has been reported in other studies of women with caesarean births (see Fisher et al. 1997). Health professionals can reduce the sense of failure that women experience by providing antenatal education about caesarean deliveries and explaining to couples that almost one in three Australian women will have a caesarean delivery. Health professionals can also assist families during the birth by explaining procedures and offering postnatal debriefing to reduce their feelings of being a failure.

4.3.4   Lack of Debriefing

Most women reported negative perceptions of their childbirth experiences and were unhappy with the lack of debriefing from health professionals after the birth. The aim of debriefing is to promote an understanding of events around the birth (Horowitz 1999) and to reduce psychological trauma (Gamble and Creedy 2004). In the literature, Waldenstrom et al. (1996) and Huack et al. (2007) found that women whose expectations of labour and birth were met were more satisfied with their childbirth experiences. Goodman and associates (2004) argued that health professionals need to provide debriefing to women to explain the circumstances around the birth and to reduce feelings of self-blame. However, in our study, most women were not given the opportunity to talk about their negative birth experiences before they were discharged from hospital. Kath discussed the need for health professionals to provide debriefing after the birth to reduce the trauma of the birth experience:

> I find that most people don't want to talk about deliveries – there's no debriefing – everyone says, "I had a horrible birth, and this and this happened. Oh, mine's worse, and mine was fine", but there's no actual debriefing.

Although the impact of a traumatic birth on maternal emotional well-being is well documented, there are only a few studies that have explored the benefit of post-partum debriefing. Cooke and Stacey (2003), in a study of women's needs in the first 2 weeks after the birth, found that 90% of primiparous women and 79% of multiparous women wanted to express their feelings about the birth with a midwife. In a systematic review of 19 publications of debriefing to reduce trauma post-delivery, Gamble and Creedy (2004) claimed that women wanted to talk about the birth with a supportive health professional. They also found that studies were inconsistent in relation to the timing and frequency of debriefing sessions; women in general wanted an understanding and sympathetic person to listen to their concerns. Gamble and Creedy (2004) argued that the ideal debriefing session would be one that provided a level of emotional support to women and included the partners.

Postnatal debriefing can be unstructured or structured and involves a discussion of women's feelings and concerns (Steele and Beadle 2003). However, there are conflicting findings in the literature as to the benefit of debriefing sessions after the birth. There are studies that have identified the benefits of debriefing on maternal adjustment and recovery (Gamble et al. 2005; Priest et al. 2003; Small et al. 2000). Gamble and colleagues (2005) assessed the intervention of a midwife-led counselling session for 348 women with trauma symptoms. The intervention group received individual counselling within 3 days of the birth and telephone support at 4–6 weeks post-partum. The counselling session included a discussion of labour management, acknowledged and validated grief and loss, offered information and enhanced social support. Gamble and colleagues (2005) claimed that 3 months post-delivery, women in the intervention group reported less symptoms of trauma, depression, stress and feelings of self-blame compared with the control group.

Some researchers have suggested that debriefing may be of no benefit to women or may cause further emotional damage. McKenzie-McHarg (2004) argues that debriefing may be damaging to women's emotional well-being if it is done too early in the post-partum period, when women are trying to process the traumatic event. McKenzie-McHarg (2004) contends that the current research neglects the psychosocial factors that contribute to trauma in the post-partum period and may explain why debriefing was not beneficial to women. This suggests the need for an individual approach to debriefing and counselling sessions. In the Cochrane Database of Systematic Reviews, Rose et al. (2006) examined 15 trials to assess the effectiveness of brief psychological debriefing for psychological distress following trauma to prevent PTSD. Rose and others (2006) argued that there is no evidence that a single session of individual psychological debriefing is useful to prevent PTSD. They concluded that debriefing reduced general psychological morbidity, depression or anxiety and that it was superior to an educational intervention.

4.4   Perceptions of PND Before Diagnosis

Couples' perceptions of PND were shaped by their personal and professional experience, media representations of PND, information accessed from parenting books and the Internet, and information received from health professionals in antenatal classes. However, the media portrayal of PND had a powerful influence over the participants' perceptions of PND as they perceived PND only in its most severe form.

4.4.1   Media Portrayals of PND

Most couples discussed the powerful nature of the media in shaping their perceptions of PND. The media portrayals of PND included television documentaries, newspaper reports and magazine articles. Postnatal depression is typically reported in the media when women either kill themselves or their children. These powerful images, combined with the lack of information about PND from antenatal classes, skewed participants' perspectives of PND before diagnosis. As a result, the participants perceived PND to be a severe disorder. Before the birth, women and their partners were clearly unaware that different degrees of severity of PND existed, adding to their confusion about the illness. The media portrayal of PND, where women either kill themselves or their children, added further confusion as it emphasised the severity of the illness. As a result, when women developed PND after the birth, they were unable to identify their experiences with PND with those portrayed in the media. One partner, Shane, discussed being aware of PND through dramatic television shows and newspaper articles where women reject or kill their children, as well as the fact that less severe cases of PND are often not reported in the media:

> My understanding was just through television stories, when the lady rejects the baby basically. When I say rejects, I've seen cases through stories where it's very dramatic, where the children actually die. I am aware of it just through the public newspapers and all that…The more severe cases because they seem to be the ones that get in the paper but we have seen other specials, I know it's not as severe as they promote it to be.

The findings from our study are supported by other studies that acknowledge the sensationalisation of mental illnesses in the media (Cutcliffe and Hannigan 2001; Francis et al. 2004; Rowe et al. 2003; Seale 2002). Seale (2002: 102), for example, described the negative and unrealistic images of mental illness depicted in the mass media:

> Considerable evidence has been gathered from a variety of countries indicating that media depictions of mental illness present unrealistically negative stereotypes of people who are out of control and prone to violence.

Newspaper articles depict the worst case scenario for PND – when women kill themselves or their children, depicting them as both mentally ill and as monsters. Cutcliffe and Hannigan (2001) argue that the depiction of mental health clients as monsters in the media creat further stigma and victimisation. The power of the mass media is even more significant if health professionals are avoiding giving couples information in case they get depressed. As a result, the media depictions of PND are not so much unrealistic, but can be insensitive and inaccurate in their portrayal of the illness as they are only showing one small slice of the condition. An examination of some of the contemporary newspaper articles over the page highlights the sensationalisation of PND in the media. Women were described as 'baby killers' before the courts determined if they were murderers or mentally ill:

> 'Mum's depression led to drowning. No jail for baby killer', when a Melbourne mother, Leanne Azzopardi, drowned her five-week-old 'miracle baby' when she wanted to stop the baby from crying (Herald Sun, December 4th, 2004).

'Teenage baby killer goes free', when Lauren Jayne Curnow, aged 17, pleaded guilty to one count of infanticide when she punched her baby to death moments after giving birth in Ballarat, Victoria (Herald Sun, April 29th 2005).

'Mother accused of killing her babies. Four murder charges'. Carol Matthey was found guilty of killing her children aged seven months, nine weeks, three months and three years in Geelong, Victoria (Herald Sun, February 25th 2005).

Another newspaper article reported that one mother was almost cheerful after killing her child:

'Mother almost "jovial" after child's death'. Sharon Anne Harrison-Taylor smothered and strangled one of her eight-month-old twins in Mt Wellington, New Zealand (New Zealand Herald, July 28th, 2005).

More sensitivity was shown by journalists when women killed themselves and not their children:

'Shooting shocks police station. Young mum's tragic death', when Ivonne Hagendoorn, policewoman and single mother, signed a gun out and shot herself minutes after she returned to work from maternity leave in Melbourne. Her baby was only four months old (Herald Sun, February 6th, 2001).

4.4.2   Lack of Information Before and After the Birth

Most couples received an insufficient amount of information about PND from health professionals before and after the birth to be able to clearly understand the condition. The participants who received little information about PND were handed only a PANDA (Post and Antenatal Depression Association) information pamphlet without a discussion of the symptoms of PND. This information was often lost in the multitude of information that was handed out in antenatal classes. Along a similar vein, Morrow and colleagues (2008) found that women, who were later diagnosed with PND in Canada, received little information about PND before the birth to be able to cope with emotional changes. The women's partners also needed information to increase their understanding of PND. However, there was a clear mismatch between the information couples needed and the information they received from health professionals before and after the birth.

Most of the first-time mothers and their partners attended antenatal classes to learn about childbirth and parenting. This is supported in the literature with studies finding that first-time mothers are more likely to attend antenatal classes compared with multiparous women (Lu et al. 2003). The focus of the antenatal classes was on the birth experience. In our study, when William was asked if he received information about PND when he attended antenatal classes, he replied:

I don't think it [PND] was brought up – it was all about how you're going to cope with the birth, and what you're going to do, and your so-called birth plan.

Early discharge from hospital also meant that women had insufficient time to receive information about PND in order to be able to understand the condition. Kelly emphasised the importance of health professionals discussing the symptoms of PND prior to discharge from hospital after the birth. She stated how important it was to let women know the number of bad days they are supposed to experience after the birth and when it would be wise to see a health professional:

> It would be helpful to be told that this can happen and you can feel like this…If they had put it more about that [PND] and say that it's normal to feel down but if you keep feeling down after so many days, you're supposed to see someone.

William also stressed the need for couples to receive information about the early warning signs of PND before leaving the hospital and the need for public education in the event that women develop PND:

> It's almost like it's taboo, and there's not a lot of public awareness. And the problem with it is if your partner's going through it, and because there's not a great deal of publicity about it you don't know about it until you're right the way – smack, bang in the middle of it. And half the battle is understanding what it is, and what affect it has on you… What are the early warning signs? If people were aware of it when they were leaving hospital that their partner could go through it [they may not feel] so much of a failure… It may even help those borderline cases from actually tipping over the edge.

Similarly, Danni discussed the lack of information she received about PND both antenatally and in the hospital, receiving information about PND only when she developed symptoms 8 months after her son's birth:

> I felt like they should make it a part of the discussion in antenatal classes and educate the men. If the men were more aware of it, of what signs to look for but they're not because like most other people they just think you're exhausted because you've got a new baby. I remember thinking at the time I can't believe they [health professionals in antenatal classes] don't do more with postnatal depression. You usually get that information [about PND] once you've bloody got it. I think in the antenatal classes they should hand out leaflets to all the clients that go through there. Maybe they should do something with the partners as well, to say well if your partner's exhibiting these signs for any length of time… I think that would help.

Sarah too suggested that:

> It's so important that people talk [about PND] and that something's done. I don't think previously there's been enough talk about it, and it's definitely something that the older generation and men don't really believe it exists because I understand that it's not just emotional, there are chemicals and things working as well. People to just sort of [not understand] hurts now, having experienced it and knowing people who have experienced it at different levels, that really hurts now – people not taking it seriously.

Marcia stated that even when she gave her partner a pamphlet about PND, he did not make the effort to read it. One year later, at the time of interview, she still carried feelings of resentment relating to her partner's refusal to read the pamphlet:

> I don't think he ever understood it, and I don't think he ever tried to understand it [laughs]. I think I said to him on the phone, I got some leaflets from PANDA, and it was all about the partner's perspective because I wanted him to understand, and he didn't even read it… I suppose I felt particularly let-down because he didn't even read the literature… whereas he might read something on how to make a million dollars in seven weeks, but to me he wouldn't read something that was so important, and important for our relationship.

The lack of information couples received about PND before diagnosis, combined with the severity of PND portrayed in the media, resulted in participants perceiving they were immune to developing PND of that severity. This is an important finding as it not only highlights the need for adequate and appropriate information to be given but also identifies that participants did not identify with the label of PND. Samantha, while aware of PND since her sister-in-law was diagnosed with the illness, still thought she was immune to developing PND:

> I remember being very aware of it [PND] but I didn't think I would be a sufferer.

One woman's partner, Luke, discussed receiving information about PND before the birth but had not considered the possibility that his partner would develop PND:

> I guess I didn't give it probably enough thought before the birth, because you never thought that it would happen to you I guess… so I really probably should have concentrated a bit more on that.

Kristina was determined not to get PND as she had considered she had always been in control in other areas of her life:

> I just knew that it wasn't anything I thought would happen to me…because I'm a very controlled person you know, and I'm very strong. Nothing's going to bother me, and I'll deal with it, and I'll get on with it… no matter what I'll always see the positive.

The need for antenatal education to improve the understanding of PND has been highlighted in previous studies. Whitton et al. (1996) stressed the importance of educating *women* (our italics) about antidepressant medication before the birth to increase their understanding and acceptance of *available treatments* (our italics). The focus on educating women, rather than couples, is reflected in the following quote by Whitton et al. (1996: 75):

> If postnatal depression is to be more readily treated, women themselves need to be more able to recognize its presence and more prepared to seek treatment. Ante-natal education is one way in which increased recognition could be achieved.

Researchers have found that women with PND receive inadequate information about PND from health professionals (Nahas et al. 1999; Skocir and Hundley 2006; Ugarriza 2002). Ugarriza (2002) found that 25 out of 30 women with PND said that if they had been more aware and knowledgeable about PND, they would have been able to cope better with the symptoms. These women were also diagnosed late with PND as a result of inadequate information received before the birth. Similarly, Nahas and colleagues (1999), in their study of Middle Eastern migrant women living in Australia, argued that women received insufficient information about PND and existing support services. These women also wanted simple, manageable and meaningful information about childbirth and parenting. Nahas et al. (1999) concluded that women would not feel like 'bad mothers' if others were more understanding of the condition.

In Australia, the Beyond Blue National Postnatal Depression Program was established in 2001 across five states including New South Wales, South Australia, Western Australia, Tasmania and Victoria (Buist et al. 2005). It is a non-profit organisation funded by national, state and territory governments (Jorm et al. 2005). The program is targeting five areas: increasing awareness, reducing stigmatisation, prevention and early intervention, training and supporting health professionals, and ongoing research (Beyond Blue 2006). The program aims to increase the awareness of PND in the community and among health professionals through education (Beyond Blue 2010). The National Postnatal Depression Program aims to identify women at-risk for antenatal or postnatal depression by screening women with the EPDS in pregnancy (26–32 weeks gestation). Women at-risk of depression are then referred to a GP, notes are made in their record, and the GP receives a copy of the National Postnatal Depression Program's management plan (Beyond Blue 2010). These women are also provided with an educational booklet, 'Emotional health during pregnancy and early parenthood'. The booklet provides information about antenatal and postnatal depression, and provides resources and contact numbers if women require further help (Beyond Blue 2010). Men also needed to be informed about PND to be able to understand the condition. Only then can the symptoms be detected early enough so that women can receive early intervention to ideally prevent or treat depressive symptoms.

4.5   Chapter Summary

The findings reported in this chapter highlight the need for support, particularly from health professionals and mothers on the journey to motherhood. The perceived lack of support can contribute to PND as women reported a sense of failure from their childbirth experiences. Significant life events in childhood, as well as pregnancy and childbirth, resulted in anxiety, depression and, in some cases, psychological trauma for many of the female participants. In childhood, the lack of emotional support from the women's mothers resulted in feelings of being unloved and rejected, and in the event of childhood sexual abuse having occurred, unprotected. The long-term effects of child sexual abuse damaged women's self-esteem, affected their relationships with others and contributed to anxiety and depressive symptoms as well as the development of PND. The number of women who were survivors of childhood sexual abuse, adult rape and domestic violence indicates a need for prenatal screening to identify women who may be particularly vulnerable to experiencing PND.

The need for support was heightened during pregnancy when most women experienced past pregnancy losses, abnormal results from antenatal testing or felt emotionally detached from their babies. At this time, women relied particularly on health professionals for informational and emotional support. Most women perceived their childbirths as traumatic when they experienced inadequate pain relief, the loss of control and the sense of failure. Some women relived their past abuse during childbirth. The lack of debriefing after the birth meant that women were unable to discuss their concerns or trauma before discharge from hospital. Women wanted to be nurtured, informed, given adequate pain relief, and wanted to feel empowered by their childbirth experiences. Instead, the women in the study felt battered, reported a sense of failure, loss of control and powerlessness as a result of their experiences. The lack of debriefing after the birth meant that issues such as trauma, the loss of control and sense of failure were not discussed before leaving the hospital. Most partners were not included to know how to support women.

There was a mismatch between the information couples needed and the information they received from health professionals before and after the birth. Most couples had a poor understanding of PND to be able to understand the condition. This fact, combined with the sensationalisation of PND in the media, meant that couples perceived PND to be a severe condition resulting in infanticide. Thus, the media was a powerful social and political influence that affected the male and female participants' understanding of PND. The focus of antenatal classes was on the birth, rather than on parenting, and meant that couples felt unprepared in their roles as parents. The next chapter will explore the psychosocial adjustment to motherhood and the challenges they faced when they became mothers and the need for support.

References

Allen, S. (1998). A qualitative analysis of the process, mediating variables, and impact of traumatic childbirth. *Journal of Reproductive and Infant Psychology, 16*, 107–131.

American Psychiatric Association. (2000). *Diagnostic and Statistical Manual of Mental Disorders, Text Revision. DSM-IV-TR* (4th revised ed.). Washington, DC: American Psychiatric Press.

Austin, M. P. (2003). Psychosocial assessment and management of depression and anxiety in pregnancy. Key aspects of antenatal care for general practice. *Australian Family Physician, 32*(3), 119–126.

Australian Institute of Health and Welfare. (2007). *The early years.* http://www.aihw.gov.au/publications/hwi/access23/access23-c02.pdf. Accessed 9 June 2010.

Bachman, G., Moeller, G., & Nenett, J. (1988). Childhood sexual abuse and the consequences in adult women. *Obstetrics and Gynecology, 71*, 631–641.

Barlow, J., Coren, E., & Stewart-Brown, S. S. B. (2006). Parent training programmes for improving maternal psychosocial health. *Cochrane Database for Systematic Reviews, 1*, No page number.

Beck, C. (2004). Birth trauma: In the eye of the beholder. *Nursing Research, 53*(1), 28–35.

Bennett, S. M., Lee, B. S., Litz, B. T., & Maguen, S. (2005). The scope and impact of perinatal loss: Current status and future directions. *Professional Psychology: Research and Practice, 36*(2), 180–187.

Beyond Blue. (2006). *What is postnatal depression?* http://www.beyondblue.org.au/index.aspx?link_id=94. Accessed 12 June 2007.

Beyond Blue. (2010). *What is postnatal depression?* http://www.beyondblue.org.au/index.aspx?link_id=94. Accessed 28 May 2010.

Birth Trauma Association. (2007). *What is birth trauma?* http://www.birthtraumaassociation.org.uk/what_is_trauma.htm. Accessed 12 June 2007.

Boyce, P. M. (2003). Risk factors for postnatal depression: A review and risk factors in Australian populations. *Archives of Women's Mental Health, 6*(Suppl.2), s43–s50.

Boyce, P., Hickey, I., & Parker, G. (1991). Parents, partners or personality? Risk factors for post-natal depression. *Journal of Affective Disorders, 21*, 245–255.

Brockington, I. (1996). *Motherhood and mental health.* Oxford: Oxford University Press.

Brown, G. R., & Anderson, B. (1991). Psychiatric morbidity in adult in-patients with childhood histories of sexual and physical abuse. *The American Journal of Psychiatry, 148*, 55–61.

Brown, G. W., & Harris, T. (1978). *Social origins of depression. A study of psychiatric disorder in women.* London: Tavistock Publications Limited.

Brown, S., Lumley, J., Small, R., & Astbury, J. (1994). *Missing Voices. The experience of motherhood.* Melbourne: Oxford University Press.

Brown, G. W., Harris, T. O., & Eales, M. J. (1996). Social factors and comorbidity of depressive and anxiety disorders. *The British Journal of Psychiatry, 168*(30), 50–57.

Buist, A. (1996). *Psychiatric disorders associated with childbirth.* Sydney: McGraw-Hill.

Buist, A. (1997). Childhood abuse, postpartum depression and parenting difficulties: A literature review of associations. *The Australian and New Zealand Journal of Psychiatry, 32*(3), 370–378.

Buist, A. (1998). Childhood abuse, postpartum depression and parenting difficulties: A literature review of associations. *The Australian and New Zealand Journal of Psychiatry, 32,* 370–378.

Buist, A. (2002). Mental health in pregnancy: The sleeping giant. *Australasian Psychiatry, 10*(3), 203–206.

Buist, A., Bilszta, J., Barnett, B., Milgrom, J., Erickson, J., Condon, J. T., et al. (2005). Recognition and management of perinatal depression in general practice. A survey of GP's and postnatal women. *Australian Family Physician, 34*(9), 787–790.

Chalmers, B. (2002). How often must we ask for sensitive care before we get it? *Birth, 29*(2), 79–82.

Church, S., & Scanlan, M. (2002). Posttraumatic stress disorder after childbirth: Do midwives play a preventative role? *The Practicing Midwife, 5,* 10–13.

Cooke, M., & Stacey, T. (2003). Differences in the evaluation of postnatal midwifery support by multiparous and primiparous women in the first two weeks after the birth. *Australian Midwifery, 16*(3), 18–24.

Cote-Arsenault, D. (1995). *Tasks of pregnancy and anxiety in pregnancy after perinatal loss: A descriptive study.* Unpublished PhD, University of Rochester, Rochester, NY.

Cote-Arsenault, D. (2003). The influence of perinatal loss on anxiety in multigravidas. *Journal of Obstetric, Gynecologic, and Neonatal Nursing, 32*(5), 623–629.

Cote-Arsenault, D. (2004). Perinatal loss. *Journal of Obstetric, Gynecologic, and Neonatal Nursing, 33*(2), 155.

Cote-Arsenault, D., & Mahlangu, N. (1999). Impact of aerinatal loss on the subsequent pregnancy and self: Women's experiences. *Journal of Obstetric, Gynecologic, and Neonatal Nursing, 28*(3), 274–282.

Cox, J. L. (1988). The life events of childbirth: Sociocultural aspects of postnatal depression. In R. Kumar & I. F. Brockington (Eds.), *Motherhood and mental illness.* London: John Wright.

Cranley, M. (1981). Development of a tool for the measurement of maternal attachment during pregnancy. *Nursing Research, 30*(5), 281–284.

Creedy, D. K., Shochet, I. M., & Horsfall, J. (2000). Childbirth and the development of acute trauma symptoms: Incidence and contributing factors. *Birth, 27*(2), 104–111.

Critchley, C. (1996, July 27th). Girls suffer more abuse. *Herald-Sun. Melbourne.*

Crockenberg, S. C., & Leerkes, E. M. (2003). Parental acceptance, postpartum depression, and maternal sensitivity: Mediating and moderating processes. *Journal of Family Psychology, 17*(1), 80–93.

Cuisinier, M., Janssen, H., de Graaw, C., Bakker, S., & Hoogduin, C. (1996). Pregnancy following miscarriage: Course of grief and some determining factors. *Journal of Psychosomatic Obstetrics and Gynaecology, 17,* 168–174.

Cutcliffe, J. R., & Hannigan, B. (2001). Mass media, 'monsters' and mental health clients: The need for increased lobbying. *Journal of Psychiatric and Mental Health Nursing, 9,* 315–321.

Czarnocka, J., & Slade, P. (2000). Prevalence and predictors of posttraumatic stress symptoms following childbirth. *The British Journal of Clinical Psychology, 39,* 35–51.

Department of Human Services. (2007). *What is child abuse?* http://hnb.dhs.vic.gov.au/children/ccdnav.nsf/FID/-D9D3DB0AF899C6E54A2567530021FEBB?OpenDocument. Accessed 12 June 2007.

Elders, M. J., & Albert, A. E. (1998). Adolescent pregnancy and sexual abuse. *Journal of the American Medical Association, 280*(7), 648–649.

Enkin, M., Keirse, M. J., Neilson, J., Crowther, C., Duley, L., Hodnett, E., et al. (2000). *A guide to effective care in pregnancy and childbirth* (3rd ed.). New York: Oxford University Press.

Finkelhor, D. (1984). *Child sexual abuse: New theory and research.* New York: The Free Press.

Fisher, J., Astbury, J., & Smith, A. (1997). Adverse psychological impact of operative obstetric interventions: A prospective longitudinal study. *The Australian and New Zealand Journal of Psychiatry, 31*, 728–738.

Fleming, J. M. (1997). Prevalence of childhood sexual abuse in a community sample of Australian women. *The Medical Journal of Australia, 166*, 65–68.

Fox, A. (2007). Miscarriage is the loss of a child, so please treat it that way. *The Australian.* http://www.theaustralian.news.com.au/story/0,20867,21314490-23289,00.html. Accessed 3 March 2007

Francis, C., Pirkis, J., Blood, W., Dunt, D., Burgess, P., Morley, B., et al. (2004). *The Australian and New Zealand Journal of Psychiatry, 38*, 541–546.

Gamble, J., & Creedy, D. K. (2004). The content and processes of postpartum counseling following a distressing birth experience: A review. *Birth, 31*, 213–218.

Gamble, J., Creedy, D. K., Moyle, W., Webster, J., Mc Allister, M., & Dickson, P. (2005). Effectiveness of a counseling intervention after a traumatic birth: A randomised controlled trial. *Birth, 32*(1), 11–19.

Goodman, P., Mackay, M. C., & Tavakoli, A. S. (2004). Factors related to childbirth satisfaction. *Journal of Advanced Nursing, 46*(2), 212–219.

Gottlieb, L. N., & Mendelson, M. J. (1995). Mothers' moods and social support when a second child is born. *Maternal-Child Nursing Journal, 23*(1), 3–14.

Harris, T. (2001). Recent developments in understanding the psychosocial aspects of depression. *British Medical Bulletin, 57*, 17–32.

Hegarty, K., Gunn, J., Chondros, P., & Small, R. (2004). Association between depression and abuse by partners of women attending general practice: Descriptive, cross-sectional survey. *British Medical Journal, 328*, 621–624.

Hennebry, G. (1998). Caring for rape survivors. *Nursing Times, 94*(17), 26–27.

Hense, A. L. (1994). Livebirth following stillbirth. In P. A. Field & P. B. Marck (Eds.), *Uncertain motherhood.* Thousand Oaks: Sage.

Herald Sun. (2001, February 6th). Shooting shocks police station. Young mum's tragic death.

Herald Sun. (2004, December 4th). Mum's depression led to drowning. No jail for baby killer.

Herald Sun. (2005, February 25th). Mother accused of killing her babies. Four murder charges.

Herald Sun. (2005, April 29th). Teenage baby killer goes free.

Hodnett, E., Gates, S., Hofmeyer, G., & Sakala, C. (2003). Continuous support for women during childbirth. *Cochrane Database of Systematic Reviews, 3*, CD003766.

Holz, K. (1994). A practical approach to clients who are survivors of childhood sexual abuse. *Journal of Nurse-Midwifery, 39*(1), 13–18.

Horowitz, M. J. (1999). *Essential papers on posttraumatic stress disorder.* New York: New York University Press.

Huack, Y., Fenwick, J., Downie, J., & Butt, J. (2007). The influence of childbirth expectations on Western Australian women's perceptions of their birth experience. *Midwifery, 23*, 235–247.

Hughes, P. M., Turton, P., Hopper, E., & Evans, C. D. H. (2002). Assessment of guidelines for good practice in psychosocial care of mothers after stillbirth: A cohort study. *Lancet, 360*, 114–118.

Hurst, S. A. (1999). Legacy of betrayal: A grounded theory of becoming demoralized from the perspective of women who have been depressed. *Canadian Psychology, 40*(2), 179–191.

Jorm, A. F., Christensen, H., & Griffiths, K. M. (2005). The impact of *beyond blue: The national depression initiative* on the Australian public's recognition of depression and beliefs about treatments. *The Australian and New Zealand Journal of Psychiatry, 39*, 248–254.

Katz-Rothman, B. (1986). *The tentative pregnancy: Prenatal diagnosis and the future of motherhood.* New York: Viking.

Kirkham, M. (1983). Labouring in the dark. Limitations on the giving of information to enable patients to orientate themselves to the likely events and timescale of labour. In J. Wilson-Barnett (Ed.), *Nursing research: Ten studies in patient care.* Chichester: Wiley.

Klier, C. M., Geller, P. A., & Neugebauer, R. (2000). Minor depressive disorder in the context of miscarriage. *Journal of Affective Disorders, 59*, 13–21.

Koo, V., Lynch, J., & Cooper, S. (2003). Risk of postnatal depression after emergency delivery. *The Journal of Obstetrics and Gynaecology Research, 29*(4), 246.

Liamputtong, P. (2007). *The journey of becoming a mother amongst women in northern Thailand.* Lanham: Lexington Books.

Lu, M., Prentice, J., Yu, S. M., Inkelas, M., Lange, L. O., & Halfon, N. (2003). Childbirth education classes: Sociodemographic disparities in attendance and the association of attendance with breastfeeding initiation. *Maternal and Child Health Journal, 7*(2), 87–93.

Mackey, M. C. (1995). Women's evaluation of their childbirth performance. *Maternal-Child Nursing Journal, 23*, 57–72.

Mackey, M. C. (1998). Women's evaluation of the labor and delivery experience. *Nursing Connections, 11*, 19–32.

Martins, C., & Gaffan, E. A. (2000). Effects of early maternal depression on patterns of infant-mother attachment: A meta-analytic investigation. *Journal of Child Psychology and Psychiatry, 41*, 737–746.

Matthey, S., Barnett, B., Howie, P., & Kavanagh, D. (2003). Diagnosing postpartum depression in mothers and fathers: Whatever happened to anxiety? *Journal of Affective Disorders, 74*, 139–147.

McKenzie-McHarg, K. (2004). Traumatic birth: Understanding predictors, triggers, and counseling process is essential to treatment. *Birth, 31*(3), 219–221.

Mercer, R. T. (1981). A theoretical framework for studying factors that impact on the maternal role. *Nursing Research, 30*, 73–77.

Milgrom, J., Martin, P. R., & Negri, L. M. (1999). *Treating postnatal depression. A psychological approach for health care practitioners.* Chichester: Wiley.

Morrow, M., Smith, J., Lai, Y., & Jaswal, S. (2008). Shifting Landscapes: Immigrant Women and Post Partum Depression. *Health Care for Women International, 29*(6), 593–617.

Mullen, P., & Fleming, J. (1998). Long term effects of child sexual abuse. *Issues in Child Abuse Prevention, 9*, 1–19.

Nahas, V. L., Hillege, S., & Amasheh, N. (1999). International exchange. Postpartum depression: The lived experiences of Middle Eastern migrant women in Australia. *Journal of Nurse-Midwifery, 44*(1), 65–74.

New Zealand Herald. (2005, July 28th). Mother almost 'jovial' after child's death.

Oakley, A. (1980). *Women confined. Towards a sociology of childbirth.* Oxford: Martin Robinson.

Oakley, A. (1992). *Social support and motherhood. The natural history of a research project.* Oxford: Blackwell.

O'Connor, T. G., Heron, J., & Glover, V. (2002). Antenatal Anxiety Predicts Child Behavioural/ Emotional Problems Independently of Postnatal Depression. *Journal of the American Academy of Child and Adolescent Psychiatry, 41*(12), 1470–1477.

Odent, M. (1984). *Birth reborn. What birth can and should be.* Random House: New York.

Palmer, R. L., Coleman, L., Chaloner, D., Oppenheimer, R., & Smith, J. (1993). Childhood sexual experiences of adults. A comparison of reports by women psychiatric patients and general practice attenders. *British Journal of Psychiatry, 163*, 499–504.

Pasternak, R. E., Reynolds, C. F., Schlernitzauer, M., Hoch, C. C., Buysse, D. J., Houck, P. R., et al. (1991). Acute open-trial nortriptyline therapy for bereavement related depression in late life. *The Journal of Clinical Psychiatry, 52*, 307–310.

Pearson, M. (1993). *Animate therapy: An introduction to sexual abuse treatment.* Maine: Technical Business Services.

Peppers, L. G., & Knapp, R. J. (1980). *Motherhood and mourning: Perinatal death.* New York: Praeger.

Priest, S. R., Henderson, J. J., Evans, S. E., & Hagan, R. (2003). Stress debriefing after childbirth. A randomised controlled trial. *Medical Journal of Australia, 178*, 542–545.

Prigerson, H. G., Shear, M. K., Jacobs, S. C., Reynolds, C. F., Maciejewski, P. K., Davidson, J. R. T., et al. (1999). Consensus criteria for traumatic grief: A preliminary empirical test. *The British Journal of Psychiatry, 174*, 67–73.

Raphael-Leff, J. (2000). Professional issues. Psychodynamic understanding: Its use and abuse in midwifery. *British Journal of Midwifery, 8*(11), 686–687.

Rhodes, N., & Hutchinson, S. (1994). Labor experiences of childhood sexual abuse survivors. *Birth, 21*(4), 213–221.

Rose, S., Bisson, J., Churchill, R., & Wessely, S. (2006). Psychological debriefing for preventing post traumatic stress disorder (PTSD). *Cochrane Database for Systematic Reviews, 1*, No page number.

Ross, L. E., Gilbert, S. E., Sellers, E. M., & Romach, M. K. (2003). Measurement issues in postpartum depression part 1: Anxiety as a feature of postpartum depression. *Archives of Women's Mental Health, 6*, 51–57.

Ross, L. E., Murray, B. J., & Steiner, M. (2005). Sleep and perinatal mood disorders: A critical review. *Journal of Psychiatry and Neuroscience, 30*(4), 247–256.

Rowe, R., Tilbury, F., Rapley, M., & O' Ferrall, I. (2003). About a year before the breakdown I was having symptoms: Sadness, pathology and the Australian newspaper media. *Sociology of Health and Illness, 25*(6), 680–696.

Rubin, R. (1967). Attainment of the maternal role. Part 1. Processes. *Nursing Research, 16*, 237–245.

Rubin, R. (1984). *Maternal identity and the maternal experience.* New York: Springer.

Ryding, E. L., Persson, A., Onell, C., & Kvist, L. (2003). An evaluation of midwives' counseling of pregnant women in fear of childbirth. *Acta Obstetricia et Gynecologica Scandinavica, 82*, 10–17.

Seale, C. (2002). *Media and health.* London: Sage.

Seguin, L., Potvin, L., St Denis, M., & Loiselle, J. (1995). Chronic stressors, social support and depression during pregnancy. *Obstetrics and Gynecology, 85*, 583–589.

Selkirk, R., McLaren, S., Ollerenshaw, A., McLachlan, A. J., & Moten, J. (2006). The longitudinal effects of midwife-led debriefing on the psychological health of mothers. *Journal of Reproductive and Infant Psychology, 24*(2), 133.

Simkin, P. (1991). Just another day in a woman's life? Women's long-term perceptions of their first birth experience. Part 1. *Birth, 18*, 203–211.

Skocir, A., & Hundley, V. (2006). Are Slovenian midwives and nurses ready to take on a greater role in caring for women with postnatal depression? *Midwifery, 22*, 40–55.

Sluckin, A. (1998). Bonding failure: 'I don't know this baby, she's nothing to do with me'. *Clinical Child Psychology and Psychiatry, 3*(1), 11–24.

Small, R., Lumley, J., Donohue, L., Potter, A., & Waldenstrom, U. (2000). Randomised controlled trial of midwife led debriefing to reduce maternal depression after operative childbirth. *British Medical Journal, 321*, 1043–1047.

Smith, M. (1998a). Childbirth in women with a history of sexual abuse (I). *The Practising Midwife, 1*(5), 20–23.

Smith, M. (1998b). Childbirth in women with a history of sexual abuse (II). *The Practising Midwife, 1*(6), 23–27.

Soet, J. E., Brack, G. A., & Dilorio, C. (2003). Prevalence and Predictors of Women's Experience of Psychological Trauma During Childbirth. *Birth, 30*(1), 36–46.

Steele, A. M., & Beadle, M. (2003). A survey of postnatal debriefing. *Journal of Advanced Nursing, 43*(2), 130–136.

Swanson, K. M. (1999). Effects of caring, measurement, and time on miscarriage impact and women's well-being. *Nursing Research, 48*, 288–298.

Sydney IVF. (2007). *Pregnancy loss.* http://www.miscarriage.com.au/basepage.cfm?id=7. Accessed 20 March 2007.

Thuet, S. K., Soule, D. J., & Fenton, L. J. (1988). The next baby: Parents' responses to perinatal experiences subsequent to a stillbirth. *Journal of Perinatology, 8*(3), 188–192.

Tilley, J. (2000). Sexual assault and flashbacks on the labour ward. *The Practising Midwife, 3*(4), 18–20.

Tsartsara, E., & Johnson, M. P. (2006). The impact of miscarriage on women's pregnancy-specific anxiety and feelings of prenatal maternal-fetal attachment during the course of a subsequent pregnancy: An exploratory follow-up study. *Journal of Psychosomatic Obstetrics and Gynecology, 27*, 173–182.

Ugarriza, D. N. (2002). Postpartum depressed women's explanation of depression. *Journal of Nursing Scholarship, 34*(3), 227–233.

Vance, J. C., Najman, J. M., Thearle, M. J., Embelton, G., Foster, W. J., & Boyle, F. M. (1995). Psychological changes in parents eight months after the loss of an infant from stillbirth, neonatal death, or sudden infant death syndrome: A longitudinal study. *Pediatrics, 96*, 933–938.

Waldenstrom, U., Borg, I. M., Ollson, B., Skold, M., & Wall, S. (1996). The childbirth experience: A study of 295 new mothers. *Birth, 23*, 144–153.

Waldenstrom, U., Hildingsson, I., Rubertsson, C., & Radestad, I. J. (2004). A negative birth experience: Prevalence and risk factors in a national sample. *Birth, 31*(1), 17–27.

Waymire, V. (1997). A triggering time: Childbirth may recall sexual abuse memories. *AWONN Lifelines, 1*(2), 47–50.

Webster, J., Linnane, J. W. J., Dibley, L. M., Hinson, J. K., Starrenburg, S. E., & Roberts, J. A. (2000). Measuring social support in pregnancy: Can it be simple and meaningful? *Birth, 27*(2), 97–101.

Westall, C. (2001). *Keeping a secret: One person's journey through pregnancy and childbirth with a history of child sexual abuse.* Unpublished minor thesis, RMIT, Bundoora

Whitton, A., Warner, R., & Appleby, L. (1996). The pathway to care in post-natal depression: Women's attitudes to post-natal depression and its treatment. *The British Journal of General Practice, 46*, 427–428.

WHO. (1993). *Introducing parents to their abnormal baby.* Geneva: Division of Mental Health.

WHO. (2000). *Women's mental health. An evidenced based review.* Geneva: WHO.

Wijma, K., Soderquist, J., & Wijma, B. (1997). Posttraumatic stress disorder after childbirth: A cross-sectional study. *Journal of Anxiety Disorders, 11*, 587–597.

Zecca, G., Gradi, E. C., Nilsson, K., Bellotti, M., Dal Verme, S., Vegni, E., et al. (2006). All the rest is normal. A pilot study on the communication between physician and patient in prenatal diagnosis. *Journal of Psychosomatic Obstetrics and Gynaecology, 27*(3), 127–130.

Chapter 5
Mothering Alone: The Adjustment to Motherhood

I think that a lot of money should be poured into programs or schools where women are given some sort of hands on experience about being a mum before they actually create a life... I think it should be compulsory. They [health professionals] should show a new mum what it's like to be a mother- the pressure, the wakeful nights, and how they manage that... and [to teach] the dads as well (Nancy).

Nancy's quote highlights the need for support from health professionals to the couples parenting skills. Becoming a mother is not just the physical act of giving birth (Barclay et al. 1997); there are profound emotional and social changes that influence women's emotional well-being (McMahon 1995; Liamputtong 2006, 2007). It was clear that the adjustment to motherhood was not a natural process. As previously stated, the biomedical model focuses on PND as a hormonal problem requiring treatment rather than women's subjective experiences. Our aim in this chapter is to highlight the challenges and complexities associated with early motherhood and the need for ongoing support.

The need for support is heightened when women become mothers as they are often isolated from other mothers in Western society (Kitzinger 1992; Putnam 2000). Support is important in the early postpartum period before women are diagnosed with PND. Early discharge from hospital can impair the amount of information, guidance and support that women receive when they become mothers (Brown et al. 2003). As a result, they attempted to learn about mothering and were often struggling to master breastfeeding and settling techniques in the privacy of their own homes with little support from others. Most women were disappointed with the amount of support they received from their partners, mothers and others. The partners worked long hours and were unable to give the women the support they needed as new mothers. Of importance, the partners' reports matched those of the women regarding the lack of support.

The lack of support from others highlighted the women's feeling of mothering alone and impacted on their personal identities. The chronic sleep deprivation contributed to women's sense of failure and affected their physical and emotional well-being.

C. Westall and P. Liamputtong, *Motherhood and Postnatal Depression: Narratives of Women and Their Partners*, DOI 10.1007/978-94-007-1694-0_5,
© Springer Science+Business Media B.V. 2011

5.1 Mothering Alone

Most women perceived they were mothering alone as they struggled with the adjustment to motherhood. In our study, most of the women were the primary caregivers for their children and undertook the bulk of domestic tasks. These findings are supported in the sociological literature that women commonly undertake more of the domestic workload than men (Busfield 1996; Mauthner 2002) and carry the ultimate responsibility of child care (Beck 1999; Pease and Wilson 1995). Instead of joyfully recalling their experiences of early motherhood, women described how they 'struggled' and could not cope with the stress and challenges of motherhood. They described motherhood as 'hard', 'exhausting' and 'thankless'. Samantha's comment highlights the relentless nature of motherhood:

> Mum would say to me, "it's hard work, you don't get paid for it, and it never stops, that's motherhood".

Diane remarked that:

> The first few weeks were just hard, because I was so tired as well after the delivery... I just started thinking, "I'm stuck with this baby, and I'm just having to feed her, and that's all I'm doing".

For Sarah, her partner also found it difficult:

> He [partner] didn't cope either, I have to say we both found it very [emphasised] different having the one [child compared] to having the two, and all that surrounded me- not working, no income, me feeling unfulfilled, and we both suffered because of that.

The importance of support for an individual's emotional well-being is well-documented. Support can improve an individual's self-esteem and sense of competence and can reduce stress (Gottlieb and Mendelson 1995). Support is multidimensional and can be broken down into perceived and actual (received) support (Gottlieb and Mendelson 1995). In the literature, there is evidence that the lack of support from others contributes to feelings of anger, loneliness and depression (Gottlieb and Mendelson 1995; Oakley 1980; Paris and Dubus 2005). The need for support is increased when women become mothers. Of importance, a positive adaptation to motherhood is related to the amount of support a woman receives in the postpartum period (Gjerdingen et al. 1991). Women need close relationships and social support to be able to cope with motherhood (Kivijarvi et al. 2004). The amount of support an individual needs stems from their own personal needs, social context and life circumstances (Gottlieb and Mendelson 1995).

In our study, many women were isolated from others as a result of moving house or when they lost their friendships at work. Three of these women commented on the isolation they experienced:

> What triggered it [PND] was moving to Melbourne because I didn't want to move... I just found it really hard. It wasn't the fact of not loving my baby, it was the lack of support and the sense of being alone. Because [my partner] had come down for a promotion, he had to work hard, so I spent a lot of my time on my own (Kris).

We moved house…but I felt a bit isolated. I gave up my job… I felt like I wasn't coping, I was exhausted…I worked three days a week in the city and I had work friends in the city. I hadn't joined the [local] community; I didn't really know anyone locally so once I was at home I felt very lonely…isolated. It was not like I had friends around with small children… my friends were all still working (Sarah).

A lot of my friends were still working, and didn't have friends with babies, so I didn't have a great support network. We don't really have family support, that's isolating too I suppose (Marcia).

Researchers have identified that women feel when they become mothers (Liamputtong and Naksook 2003; McVeigh 1997; Tarkka 2003). McVeigh (1997) found that women felt isolated from others when there was insufficient support in the postpartum period. Tarkka (2003) argued that the more isolated women were after the birth, the more incompetent they felt as mothers as they were unable to tap into support networks. Liamputtong and Naksook (2003) found that Thai women were socially isolated from other mothers in Australia due to their culture and trying to adjust to a new land.

One of the most influential researchers in the area of maternal adjustment, Mercer (2004), conducted a synthesis of qualitative research that explored the transition to motherhood for primiparous and multiparous women. From these studies, Mercer (2004) contends that there are four key stages in the process of establishing maternal identity: (a) commitment, attachment and preparation (pregnancy); (b) acquaintance, learning and physical restoration (first 2–6 weeks after the birth); (c) moving towards a new normal (2 weeks to 4 months); and (d) achievement of the maternal identity (around 4 months). Mercer (2004) states that the time for achieving the last three stages is variable and influenced by maternal and infant variables and the social environmental context, which is particularly relevant to our study. The stage, 'Moving toward a new normal' becomes predominant when the mother 'learns the nuances of her baby's behaviour' (Mercer 2004: 231). These stages may overlap, and physical recovery may not occur within 6 weeks postpartum (Mercer 2004).

In our study, the adjustment to motherhood was also affected by women's physical well-being. Physical restoration took longer than 6 weeks for some women as they experienced bladder problems and abscesses, and had infected tears and episiotomies. In general, women achieved their maternal identities 1–2 years after the birth when they had largely resolved their depressive symptoms, felt comfortable in their own bodies, felt attached to their babies and felt competent in their roles as mothers. For most women in the study, the adjustment to motherhood was a lengthy process as women were struggling with depressive symptoms. Erin's adjustment to motherhood was shadowed by symptoms of PND that started immediately after the birth. She experienced a 12-month adjustment to motherhood which was complicated by the death of her mother when she was 6 months pregnant:

I remember sitting on the couch with a girlfriend, our kids were twelve months old…and I said to her, "I think I've only just come to terms with this motherhood thing". Whether that was only just coming out of my depression…that's how long it took me to wrap [emphasised] my mind around my new life.

Several studies explored the adjustment to motherhood for women with PND (Beck 2002a; Berggren-Clive 1998; Brown et al. 1994; Buultjens and Liamputtong 2007; Fowles 1998; Holopainen 2002; Mauthner 1999). Beck (2002a) conducted a metasynthesis of 18 qualitative studies of PND published between 1990 and 1999. The studies included a total of 309 women from the United States, United Kingdom, Australia and Canada. The four main themes that emerged were: incongruity between expectations and the reality of motherhood (conflicting expectations, shattered dreams, fear of being labelled and cultural context); spiralling downwards (anxiety, overwhelmed, obsessive thinking, anger, cognitive impairment, isolation/loneliness, guilt and contemplating on harming self); pervasive loss (loss of control, loss of self, loss of relationship and loss of voice) and making gains (surrendering, struggling to survive and reintegration and change).

5.2   Unmet Expectations of Support

For most women, the reality of motherhood was far different to their expectations, particularly in relation to support. The unmet expectations of support resulted in disappointment, loss of self-esteem and isolation from others and disillusionment with the motherhood role. Wilkinson and Mulcahy (2010) also found that women with PND have inadequate social support. Multiparous women reported that there was an assumption that they were experts, and they felt guilty when they were unable to spend as much time with older children. Erin discussed the expectation with her second child:

> There is an expectation when you have your second child that everyone says, "It's so much easier the second time around". And yes it is in a lot of ways- you're more skilled, you're more confident as a mother. But that expectation is that you should be able to do this now, you're cruising now.

The disparity between the expectations and realities of motherhood is well-documented in the literature for women with PND (Barclay and Lloyd 1996; Berggren-Clive 1998; Buultjens and Liamputtong 2007; Lauer-Williams 2001; McVeigh 1997; Podkolinski 1998; Rubin 1984; Tammentie et al. 2004). Tammentie and colleagues (2004) found that parents, particularly mothers, strove for perfection; perceived their infants had tied them down and had high expectations of family life. Berggren-Clive (1998: 111) aptly used the term 'the disillusionment with motherhood' as women experienced conflict with the expectations of themselves as the perfect mother. Oakley (1980) argued that if the reality experienced is different to women's expectations, there is a marked impact upon self-esteem. McVeigh (1997) claimed that women expected to cope and felt alone when they became mothers. The literature supports the notion that the reality of motherhood was different to expectations for women diagnosed with PND in Australia (Buultjens and Liamputtong 2007; Morgan et al. 1997; Nahas et al. 1999; Nahas and Amasheh 1999) and overseas (Berggren-Clive 1998; Mauthner 1995, 1999; Nicolson 1990, 1999; Wood et al. 1997).

5.2.1   Feeling Unprepared

Most couples discussed feeling unprepared with their first babies despite attending antenatal classes, meeting with health professionals, accessing internet sites and reading books. Couples typically received adequate information about the birth but inadequate information about parenting. As discussed in Chapter 4, there was insufficient information given to couples in antenatal classes about PND and parenting for them to feel competent in their roles as parents. This finding is consistent with previous research (Nolan 1997; Underdown 1998).

As a result of feeling unprepared, most women were anxious and overwhelmed in their new roles as mothers. Multiparous women were more likely to feel prepared as they were aware of infant demands, although they also had the added expectation of knowing what to do if problems arose, particularly if the baby was unsettled. The notion of feeling unprepared for first-time motherhood has been reported extensively in the literature (Barclay et al. 1997; Brockington 1996; Brown et al. 1994; Costello 1976; Crouch and Manderson 1993; Kiehl and White 2003; Mercer 2004; Morrow et al. 2008; Oakley 1980; Pridham et al. 1994; Rogan et al. 1997; Rubin 1984), regardless of the age and emotional well-being of the mother. Rogan and associates (1997) argued that first-time mothers felt unprepared and overwhelmed in the early weeks of motherhood as they faced new and unexpected challenges. The feeling of being unprepared contributed to women's feelings of emotional upheaval and a disturbed sense of self (Rogan et al. 1997). None of the women in their sample were diagnosed with PND.

Researchers have argued that it is important for couples to attend antenatal classes to prepare them for birth and parenting (Pridham et al. 1994). Several studies have found that women who were inadequately prepared for motherhood were more likely to feel inadequate as mothers (Brockington 1996; Kiehl and White 2003; Mercer 2004). In our study, all of the couples attended antenatal classes with their first babies. However, as previously discussed, there was a mismatch between the information they needed and the information they received. Luke attended antenatal classes with his wife, Monica. He discussed the numerous changes after the birth that impacted on their confidence as parents:

> We both went to the antenatal classes and went through all that training, and I don't know if we weren't listening but we found it so [emphasised] difficult that first twelve months. It was incredibly difficult, and I'm quite sure that a big element of it [PND] was the fact that we weren't really aware of the changes in our lives… You go from a completely free and easy sort of life, and sleep as long as you like… to something where you're twenty-four hours on demand sort of thing, and it's quite draining. That constant drain- and that significant change in your life had a big impact as well.

Nancy felt unprepared when her first baby was born and did not have time to bond with her baby as she was overwhelmed with the responsibility of having a child. Her words, 'please tell me what to do', convey a sense of helplessness and urgency to learn about mothering:

> I don't know what I was feeling but it wasn't an instant bond. The first time was an overwhelming realisation of the responsibility of having a child, and while I was coming to

terms with those feelings [laughs] I didn't have any time to bond. So it was immediate, "please tell me what to do as quickly as possible so I can have order in my life again"… Look I didn't know what to expect as a mother, no-one really tells you, it's very hands-on. So it was a shock to my system with the first [child] and a double-shock to my system when I had two [children] so close in age- seventeen months is the difference between the two [children].

Tara's account is typical of the first-time mothers interviewed as she felt unprepared in her role as a mother despite accessing information from books and health professionals.

I couldn't believe she was my baby… It was very hard to link the pregnancy and this whole expectation that totally consumed me. To the fact that now in front of me is this baby. They're just very different things. I'm sure that's part of the whole postnatal depression experience and the whole just adjusting to motherhood thing, because they're just very different experiences… But when it actually happens it's just different. You just think, I'm not prepared for this. I'm not prepared for this. What do I do now?… Yet I'd prepared, I'd read everything I could read, I'd spoken to everyone I could speak to, and bought everything I could buy… Suddenly I didn't know what to do.

Ellie also spoke about the difficult adjustment to motherhood, feelings of disappointment and sense of being unprepared after the birth. She reflected back on her experience and her expectation of being able to cope with motherhood:

I had no idea of what to expect first time around with a new baby. I thought I'd be going for coffees with girlfriends, mother's group, having lunch, going shopping. Yeah, and was faced with quite a reality shock… I thought this is very foreign. It didn't come naturally. It was all going pear-shaped. It wasn't how I'd planned, and being a planner, and an organised person I thought that… it would have gone the way I wanted and obviously when it didn't I was really disappointed.

Women were also disappointed when they received a lack of emotional support from their mothers.

5.2.2   Relationship with Mother

As women felt unprepared for motherhood, they turned to their mothers for support. Despite a less-than-ideal mother-daughter relationship for most women in our study, women's relationships with their mothers were central to their stories. They described their maternal relationship as 'absent', 'superficial', 'distant','not terrific', 'non-existent', involving 'not much communication', a'lack of relationship','dutiful' and 'not close'. As a result, most women had difficulty accessing the emotional support, practical help, mothering skills and reassurance they needed for their sense of competence and self-esteem. Most women also described their mothers as 'selfish', 'unhappy', 'angry', 'used guilt to control', 'never told me she loved me', 'never praised', 'in the victim role', 'distorted thinking','highlights the negative' and'depressed'.

In our study, most of the women had mothers who were diagnosed with PND or depression. This finding is congruent with the literature that women with a family history of mental illness are at increased risk of developing PND (American

Psychiatric Association 2000; Mauthner 2002; Milgrom et al. 1999). One mother of one of the participants was on antidepressant medication for over 30 years. Although women often shared a depressive experience with their mothers, because of their emotionally distant relationship, they were unable to discuss their experience of PND with them. As Beatrice explained:

> I don't know that I feel particularly close to her…we're not mates like some mothers and daughters are… Mum's had acute depression, probably had postnatal depression I suspect, although it's not the sort of thing we can talk about.

Tara commented on the lack of maternal support that other mothers in her PND support group experienced:

> I know when I was in a group for postnatal depression I noticed lots of people didn't have support, and particularly didn't have their mothers around. I found that really interesting that there was no motherly support- whether it was there wasn't a good relationship there or there was a distance involved, physical distance, where they couldn't travel to each other- there seemed to certainly be a pattern there of not having support from a mother… I remember being very upset one day with postnatal depression, totally overwhelmed by it all, and she [Rose] had been crying and crying and crying- you know one of those sort of days. I called my mum in tears and said, "I'm not coping", and all she could say was, "well that's motherhood dear". That was it and I think I hung up quite promptly and called somebody else.

Kim spoke about the emotionally distant relationship she had with her mother. In this relationship, she was unable to receive the emotional support she needed to feel confident to help her adjust to motherhood as she perceived her mother as 'sarcastic'. She explained:

> You don't tell her that emotional stuff because she just twists that and uses it against you. You know it's your fault, I told you so, all that, [she's very] sarcastic.

Mary expected her mother to visit her in the hospital when she gave birth to her second baby. Mary felt abandoned and extremely disappointed when her mother who lived so close to the hospital chose not to visit her:

> I just burst into tears, and she [the nurse] is like, "What's wrong?" [I said] "My mum hasn't come to visit me"… "Where does she live?" "About twenty minutes away". She [said], "well, you can't worry about that, you're a mum now and you just worry about your child". That's all the advice I got.

Similarly, Kyle reflected back on the disappointment his wife, Lisa, experienced when she received insufficient support from both her mother and sister after the birth. He confronted Lisa's mother to access support:

> She was very disappointed in her mother's behaviour- her mother's lack of support… Lisa had an idea that she would be more supported- by her mum particularly, and it didn't happen. I actually rang her mother up after four months and said, "You'd better get down here, Lisa's not managing, and you're not giving her any support. She wants you [emphasised]. You're her mother, whether you get along with her or not has nothing to do with it. She wants you. She needs you. I go to work"… She was also a bit disappointed with her sister. It's not that they weren't there- they weren't listening to her. They weren't resonating and picking up on her quiet calls for support and help.

The death of Erin and Danni's mothers had a major impact on their emotional well-being:

> My mum died at the time I became a mother, so I was dealing with looking at her and her life, and then looking at myself as a mother, and my childhood. So it just brought it all home in a really big rush for me. … I lost my mum when I was six months pregnant, so obviously that was tragic, awful… I remember sitting in the bath probably half-way through my mum's hospital stay, and I felt like I was going to have a nervous breakdown… I remember thinking, just hold it together. I don't want this to affect this baby. So I remember thinking when mum died, I'm doing really well, she's helping me, I've got it together, until she [my daughter] was born (Erin).

> I think probably even from the age of ten when my mother died I reckon if someone had clinically looked at me then they would have found that I was seriously, seriously depressed as a ten year old child after her death because I found her. So for so many years after her death every time I closed my eyes I'd see her dead. I think really looking back on it; I think from a young child I was really prone to bouts of depression (Danni).

In the literature, there is evidence that children of mothers with PND have higher rates of insecure attachment than children of non-depressed mothers (Martins and Gaffan 2000). Maushart (1997) claimed that an emotional disconnection with women's own mothers means that the practical skills of mothering are not passed down from mother to daughter. Practical support has been identified as important for preparing for the demands and challenges of motherhood (Milgrom et al. 1999). In our study, the lack of emotional support and practical help from their own mothers resulted in the loss of self-esteem and may have influenced their ability to cope with motherhood. Researchers have found that emotional support and reassurance are both important for self-confidence and self-esteem (Barclay et al. 1997; Gottlieb and Mendelson 1995; Hart 1981).

The women who had distant relationships with their mothers wanted to be more nurturing than their own mothers after the birth. They expressed a conscious desire to mother their children differently. Kim stated that her mother 'sat there like a visitor' when she visited her in hospital shortly after the birth. Kim discussed the lack of support from her mother and her decision to be more affectionate with her child:

> I just felt like she just rejected [my daughter], she wouldn't hold her, wouldn't give her a cuddle or if she did it was for like thirty seconds and then she'd pass her on. A lot of other mums are around and my mum probably came twice in the first three months and when she did she sat there like a visitor, so she wasn't supportive like that at all… I can learn from how she mothered me, I don't have to mother that way. I can show more affection to [daughter], that it's okay for [partner] to give me a kiss in front of the kids, that's fine.

The mother-daughter relationship has been neglected in much of the recent literature investigating the transition to motherhood for women with PND. Mauthner's (2002) 10-year research project was published in a book entitled, *The Darkest Days of My Life: Stories of Postpartum Depression*. Mauthner (2002) found that women wanted to be independent and separate to their own mothers after the birth of their babies. The findings from our study differed as women expected and craved the emotional and practical support from their mothers and did not want to be separated emotionally from them. Mauthner (2002) claimed that women's relationships with their own mothers were central to their stories, even when their relationships were emotionally distant. Similarly, Mercer (1985) argued that a woman's own mother was the most important support for her in the mothering role. Along a similar vein, Nelson (2003) found that support from a woman's own mother was important because women need to talk about their concerns, questions and conflicts.

The lack of support from women's own mothers after the birth has been documented in the literature (Buultjens and Liamputtong 2007; Mauthner 2002; Mercer 1981; Morrow et al. 2008). There is evidence in the literature that women who have a poor relationship with their own mothers are at risk of developing depression (Buultjens and Liamputtong 2007; Chaffin et al. 1996; Mauthner 2002; Milgrom et al. 1999; Tomison 1996).

5.2.3   Learning to Be a Mother

In our study, learning about mothering was more difficult when women had insufficient support from female role models and health professionals, making the transition to motherhood more difficult. The absence of support set women up for failure as they did not feel competent in their maternal roles. As women received insufficient support from female role models and health professionals, they tried to learn about motherhood from trial and error and from books and the internet rather than from other mothers and health professionals. Learning from trial and error is harder than learning from other mothers as it requires more time and patience.

Motherhood is learned by observing female role models (Hart 1981; Bergum 1986; Nelson 2003) and through support offered by others. In the literature, it is well-documented that women are faced with a considerable learning curve when they become mothers (Barclay et al. 1997; Buultjens and Liamputtong 2007; Mercer 2004; Rubin 1961). In their research, Barclay and colleagues (1997) used the category 'working it out' to encompass the learning associated with first-time motherhood as women observed friends and relatives to see what worked. The process of 'working it out' was individual and was dependent on maternal factors (lack of self-confidence) and infant characteristics (infant temperament).

Samantha shared the sentiments of many women participants that motherhood was a time of learning and was a difficult adjustment. She felt the pressure to do 'everything right' and, at the same time, was confused by the information she was receiving. Samantha's quote highlights the need for support and guidance from health professionals:

> We've got to learn to do formula, we've got to learn to get her to sleep; we've got to do controlled crying but when does that start? You hear all these things but you don't know exactly at what point of time, and you want to do everything right. Everything you want to do right, by the book, how they've taught you. Be aware for this, be aware for that, don't put them in your bed, [and] don't do this with SIDS.

Women sought out role models to observe their behaviour with their infants and to watch how other mothers were coping with motherhood. However, critical comments by others meant that women were unable to access the support they needed. Researchers have found that unhelpful support, such as critical comments from others, may undermine a woman's self-confidence as a mother (Leff et al. 2000). The dialogue in the focus group with the male partners emphasises the need for women to learn about motherhood and the paradox of women being cruel to other women:

> Nick: What I've found is actually women are quite cruel to women, that's my view. The other mums, they're not as sensitive, and don't think about what they're saying. They can be quite cruel and say, "I did it. Why can't you?" [Other mums have] no empathy… I just notice this even in everyday life women can be pretty cruel to each other [everyone agreeing].
>
> Nathan: "It was hard for me, it should be hard for you too!" [Everyone laughing]… It's sort of like a retribution type of thing in a way.
>
> Michael: They [midwives] just see it every day, every day they live and not like individuals trying to learn.

Similarly, Erin discussed the enormous learning curve associated with becoming a mother and the need for support from health professionals. Rather than sugar coating motherhood, she stressed the need for health professionals to teach mothers important skills to prepare them for motherhood:

> I remember thinking, rather than those bullshit antenatal classes they should put you in something like the mother-baby unit, and teach you how to be a mother- teach you settling skills…tell you how bad it's going to be you know, rather than sugar coat it, because that's how you feel…You've got these romanticised ideals of how it's going to be, and you're living it and you think, hang on a minute, this is not right! But they [health professionals] should give you the reality check like I got in the mother-baby unit.

Learning to be a mother has been well-documented in the literature (Kivijarvi et al. 2004). Maternal sensitivity behaviour is an important aspect of mothering as it requires women to recognise the infant's cues and respond to them (Kivijarvi et al. 2004). When women respond to their infants, there is a mutual pleasure and enjoyment they both share (Bromwich 1976). Mead (1934) describes four components to role learning: play (practice in role acquisition), fantasy (silent rehearsal of roles), empathy (identification with another) and copying (mimicking the actions of others). Copying requires the role model to be present so the behaviour can be mimicked (Mead 1934). In our study, the lack of these four components of role learning contributed to women's low self-esteem and the loss of self.

5.3   Multiple Losses Leading to the Loss of Self

The main loss that women experienced that encompassed most of the other losses was the loss of self. Women faced multiple losses when they became mothers, such as the loss of work relationships, the temporary loss of careers and the loss of independence. When women were unable to meet the demands of motherhood, they experienced the loss of self-confidence and self-esteem. The notion of loss of self was influenced by women's interaction and observation of other mothers in society. Carson and Arnold (1996) contend that our sense of self is defined by others in our social environment, such as our family and reference groups. In our study, women lost their sense of self when they felt different to other mothers, lost their previous identities and struggled with the adjustment to motherhood. As a result, women experienced a sense of failure and hid behind a facade to hide their identities. These findings are supported in the literature by Keating-Lefler and Wilson (2004), who argued that women lost their identities when they became mothers – who they were and who they would become. Hurst (1999) also found that depressed women experienced the loss of self and the loss of identity. Buultjens and Liamputtong (2007) claimed that women with PND experience the loss of self-esteem. Similar to the findings by Rogan and associates (1997), many women in our study experienced a loss of self-confidence, loss of self-esteem and a negative perception of themselves as mothers. Appleby et al. (1997) contended that negative attitudes to the self were associated with PND. Georgia described the loss of self and low self-esteem she experienced as a mother when she gave up her career for motherhood:

> I don't think I was prepared for that loss, the loss of knowing who I was, and I felt a tremendous loss of self in terms of motherhood… I had to go through this huge personal thing of re-discovering who I was, and what I discovered was if you take away my work, and all these other little crutches to believe I'm a person then I don't cope particularly well.

Most women discussed facing numerous changes, many of which they had difficulty accommodating when they became mothers. These findings are supported by other researchers (see Nicolson 1999; Rogan et al. 1997). Nicolson (1999) found that poor mental health occurred when women were unable to adapt and grow with the changes associated with motherhood. Tara reflected on the numerous changes and challenges that occurred with motherhood and the loss of self-esteem she experienced in her new role as a mother:

> Your role totally changes in life, and suddenly you're seen by everyone as a mother, and that's a very different thing to being seen as an independent woman who works… All of a sudden you don't work and you don't have that identity of being a co-worker- those relationships they've gone, or at least on hold… You think who am I? If this is my only role and I'm not good at it, so it's that belief that, I'm not good at it, and that's now who I am… What you used to do every day changes. You don't go to work anymore, you just have a whole new set of expectations and even your own body is different, your relationship with your partner [and] your own body is different, everything's different. Suddenly you've got no pelvic floor muscles, you've got a sagging stomach and these huge breasts, you don't even feel like you're in your own body and I think that's a huge thing.

The loss of self for women with PND has been reported extensively in the sociological literature (Appleby et al. 1997; Beck 1992, 1993; Beck 2005; Berggren-Clive 1998; Dalton 1996; Dix 1987; Hurst 1999; Keating-Lefler and Wilson 2004; Mauthner 1999; Nicolson 1990, 1999; Nims 1996; Semprevivo 1996; Wood et al. 1997). Mauthner (1999) claimed that women experience multiple losses when they become mothers, such as the loss of identity, autonomy, independence, power and paid employment. Beck (2005) argued that the loss of self was an important component of PND and included it as a dimension on the

Postpartum Depression Screening Scale. In the literature, loss has been reported as a key feature of depression (Brown et al. 1995; Dalton 1996; Nicolson 1990, 1999). While Dalton (1996: 51) described depression as a 'disease of loss', Brown (1998) stated that loss in itself was not enough to cause depression but, combined with on-going difficulties, was enough to contribute to feelings of hopelessness and depression.

Researchers have argued that childbirth and early motherhood experiences can be explained by models of loss and bereavement (Barclay and Lloyd 1996; Berggren-Clive 1998; Driscoll 1990; Nicolson 1990, 1999; Oakley 1980). Rogan and colleagues (1997) claimed that the losses associated with motherhood were associated with grieving and sometimes resentment. Brown, Bifulco and Harris (1987) stated that loss is usually involved if it is connected to a person's role as it is associated with the loss of identity. The loss of self has been reported in studies of non-depressed women (Keating-Lefler and Wilson 2004; Rogan et al. 1997). However, what was different for the women in our study was the loss of self-esteem and perception of themselves as bad mothers when they interacted or observed other mothers.

5.3.1 Feeling Different to Other Mothers

The majority of women felt they were different to other mothers in the early postpartum period and before they were diagnosed with PND. Unfortunately, these women missed the opportunity for interaction with other mothers because they had personal feelings of being 'bad mothers' as they had difficulty settling and/or breast feeding their babies. Women's perceived feelings of being different to other mothers resulted in feelings of isolation from others and the lack of support. This feeling of isolation and the lack of support for women with PND was reported by Nahas and associates (1999). The notion of feeling different to other mothers has not been documented in the literature prior to the onset of PND and is an important finding as it has implications for detecting early symptoms of PND.

In our study, when women felt different to other mothers, they became isolated and had difficulty learning from other mothers. The social disconnection also meant that emotional, practical and informational support was not accessible from other mothers. Rather, women felt judged by other mothers when they tried to access support. Spending time with other mothers increased their feelings of inadequacy and resulted in negative perceptions of themselves as 'bad mothers'. When this support was not forthcoming and when women were later diagnosed with PND, they turned to other depressed women for advice and support. Monica's first-time mother's group added to her feelings of inadequacy and depression as she felt judged when she was unable to settle her baby. She described the isolation she experienced as a result of dropping out of the group:

> I know my mother's group started quite late, and I know I wasn't on medication when that started. And I know that probably pushed me over to be honest, which sounds terrible. I sat

in a room with thirteen other women whose babies were quiet, and who actually looked at me and said, "Why can't you settle your baby? Have you tried this? Have you tried that?"… And the maternal and child health nurse knew exactly what I'd been through, and she would try and come and help me, but I couldn't stand sitting there for two hours…I just didn't go after that. It was too hard. Once we stopped meeting in the confines of the health centre I didn't go, and I regret that now because I don't have that network of people with kids the same age…but at the time it was the right thing to do because it made me worse.

Similarly, Maria had difficulty fitting in with the new parents' group. She discussed her feelings of inadequacy when she attended the group. The group did enable her to compare her emotional well-being with other mothers but was unhelpful as others were unable to understand her difficulties with motherhood. Maria reflected back on her feeling of being different to other mothers in the new mothers' group:

All the other mums seemed to be having no problems. She [baby] would cry all day, and they'd say, "Just stick her in the rocker". I didn't even know what a rocker was. At that point [the maternal and child health nurse] said, "Oh, that's nothing". They all said, "Oh, that's nothing to get depressed about". It was a big deal. And I look back now, and I know that yes, when you have PND something as simple as that is such a big drama, and a big deal- just too overwhelming. And of course then it's not a problem. It was like everyone was saying, "No, no, that's just normal. That's just fine". I couldn't work out why I couldn't cope with normal.

Even offers of help were misconstrued as Tara explained:

If someone offered to help that would mean that they thought I couldn't cope and I was really bad at being a mother.

In our study, an important finding was that women experienced the stigma of being different to others, and this occurred in early motherhood and before the diagnosis of PND. Bridget compared herself to other mothers to gauge how she was coping with motherhood. She described herself being on a different wavelength to other mothers in the new mothers' group and 'hinting' that something was wrong, but other mothers were unable to understand:

I thought if this is life it's pretty crap. I just thought with all these mums if this is what we're going through, I thought I'm just not coping well with it. You'd see other people in mother's group when I used to even half-hint they didn't seem to be on that same wave length and I thought I'm not coping as well… I just thought I wasn't finding it as easy.

Tara told us that:

I was feeling very judged- I was feeling like everyone was judging what sort of a mother I was. I was very defensive so I wasn't opening up to people because I didn't want to say, "Hey look I'm having a hard time… " I was very guarded about all of that- I wasn't open to people helping me in a practical way or in an emotional way, so whatever structures we'd set up were just useless really.

The notion of feeling different to other mothers in our study contrasts findings of Barlow and Cairns (1997) who argued that first-time mothers find it beneficial to spend time with other new mothers for reassurance and to reduce feelings of inadequacy. Similar findings were reported in a qualitative American study by Paris and Dubus (2005); common themes included isolation, loneliness and disconnection from other mothers. In addition to these themes, our study suggests that stigma occurred in early motherhood and before the diagnosis of PND. There is evidence in the literature that individuals with depression feel inferior to others (Allan and Gilbert 1997; Birchwood et al. 2000; Eriksen and Kress 2005; Gilbert and Allan 1998; Goffman 1961, 1963, 1971, 1972; Kauffman 2003; Smith 2002; Thompson et al. 2004; WHO 1999).

Stigma occurs when individuals perceive themselves as different to others. Goffman (1971) discusses the link between an individual feeling different to others and the alienation from interaction. The notion of stigma is related to feelings of insecurity and inferiority women experienced as mothers. Goffman (1963: 15) writes extensively about the stigma of mental illness and defined stigma as 'an undesired differentness from what we had anticipated'. Eriksen and Kress (2005) suggest that stigmatised individuals perceive themselves as weak and carry feelings of self-blame, shame and isolation as they feel excluded from society. Goffman (1963) claims that stigma creates feelings of inferiority, insecurity, anxiety and depression. Stigma can deprive people of their dignity and interferes with individuals participating fully in society (WHO 1999). In our study, this finding was a later barrier for women getting treatment for their depressive symptoms. Some women also experienced a delayed attachment to their babies, which also contributed to the feeling of being different to other mothers.

5.3.2 Delayed Bonding with Baby

The majority of women in our study reported a delay in bonding either initially or when they were discharged from hospital, and a large number of these women experienced perinatal losses (see also Chapter 1). Although the average length of time for delayed bonding was 3–4 months, one woman reported a significant delay with bonding for 13 years. Most women reported a delayed attachment to their babies starting either immediately after the birth or within months after the birth, and this detachment lasted for months or years. Women's reported lack of attachment to their babies threatened their self-confidence and self-esteem. These women commonly talked about feeling 'too tired to bond' with their infants as they had little opportunity for rest or respite. Buultjens, Robinson and Liamputtong (2008) found that the attachment that women with PND had with their infants was tarnished by their depression. Wilkinson and Mulcahy (2010) claim that women with PND report reduced attachment to their infant.

Multiparous women in our study were able to compare their experiences of bonding with their babies and were able to articulate a noticeable difference in the attachment. Beatrice was one of the multiparous women who noticed a distinct difference in the attachment between her first and second babies. It took Beatrice thirteen years to attach to her son because of the behavioural difficulties he experienced from childhood into adolescence. She distanced herself from her first pregnancy because of her past miscarriage and was also more attached to her baby when she found out she was a girl. Beatrice reflected back on her experience with bonding:

I was really conscious of something being amiss in the whole early process with [my son]. With [my daughter], as I did with [my son], I picked them up and put them to the breast and cuddled them. With [my daughter] I rubbed my face around her face and I sniffed her head and kissed her. Maybe it was the smell of her and wanting to know what she smelled like, it must have been a hormonal, emotional surge and when you think bonding you can almost hear it [laughs], click, yes we bonded. With [my son], especially looking back on it, [bonding] didn't happen the first time.

Marcia described loving her son and meeting his needs but not feeling an 'emotional connection' to him. She described attachment as a 'warm, fuzzy feeling' and discussed her disconnection with her first baby when she was diagnosed with PND:

I was diagnosed with postnatal [depression] after Carl, so I don't think I connected with him... for quite a few weeks really. I mean not that I wasn't meeting his needs, I think more of an emotional connection, I'm supposed to love this baby. I did [love him] but it was just not that warm, fuzzy feeling.

The delayed attachment to the baby also occurred when women were unable to settle their infants, and this resulted in their personal sense of failure. In general, women believed they would have a stronger bond with their infants if their babies were more settled. Maria reflected on her feelings of having difficulty connecting with her baby. As a result, she perceived herself as a 'failure' when her child was constantly unsettled:

I felt like I should love this baby, and I did but I wouldn't let myself really feel it. She didn't want to feed. We just didn't gel. She just puked [vomited] all the time, and cried all the time. Nothing I seemed to do [helped to] settle her. I just felt like I had no effect on her. I used to say to [my husband] that I almost regretted having her, because we didn't seem to connect [pause]. When she was a screamer...and one that didn't sleep...there was just this whole sense of failure that just got drummed in.

Women commonly reported meeting the physical needs of their infants but not their own emotional needs:

I said to Tim last night, "Carl didn't smile for a long time", and that was probably my lack of communication to him, and interaction with him. I think I met his physical needs well, but didn't bond and speak to him a lot, and it was probably a pretty quiet time (Marcia).

All I could manage were his basic needs, he had food and his nappies were clean. I didn't shower myself for four days, I didn't care. I felt nothing when I looked at him, nothing. It was just this parasite that was living off me and I was still breast feeding him so he was sucking the life out of me... I didn't want anything to do with him (Danni).

For some women, the sex of the baby was a disappointment and a 'shock':

I did cry when I found out that Tom was a boy, because my husband had wanted a little girl (Georgia).

When he was born and they said, "He's a little boy", because I honestly believed he was a little girl, and it was a little boy. I think I was in shock (Barbara).

It was a shock because he was a boy, I just thought I was having a girl [laughs]... It just took a while to get used to after thinking for all this time I was having a girl (Ursula).

Because of their emotional stage, older children sometimes took on the parenting role:

Vicky was so good because she'd come and give me a cuddle and say "it's okay mummy"... she knew that I was upset because I was crying (Ursula).

I remember Kylie was doing something... and I actually pushed her down the stairs and I scared myself. And the same day Carol was crying and I was sitting down there and she was on the floor in front of me and I screamed at her "will you stop crying?" Bernadette came running down and said "don't yell at her mummy, she's only little, she can't help crying". I can honestly say I would have killed my children, I really would have at that point... I don't think I ever told Trevor [my husband] (Lyn).

Beatrice was the only participant who expressed concerns about her son's emotional well-being:

When Danielle was born I was having such enormous trouble with Ethan because he did actually want to kill (emphasised) her which made life very difficult. I had to actually put a really high lock on her bedroom door so I could answer the phone and go to the toilet, and I was really frightened what he might do to her ... I saw him standing over her with scissors one day and I was terrified. [At two years of age] Ethan started seeing the psychiatrist (Beatrice).

Later in the interview she stated:

[At school] he really hurt other children, he was violent and drew blood, did all sorts of things to other kids or broke things, he's broken seven or eight doors and three or four windows in his life, it's probably about nine now including his own.

A small number of women like Samantha and Sarah took out their anger and frustration on their children:

I was being nasty to her, probably bordering on being really cruel to her verbally. She's a smart girl; she knew what was going on. I would want to just reduce her to tears, that was my aim.... because that's how I felt (Samantha).

I shouted at her and then I felt horrible about that, and probably felt guilty, you always feel guilty. Probably it did make me feel less love and not as much affection towards Fay because she was the cause of it all. Then realising that she's not the cause of it all, I'm the cause of it all, and how that made me feel about myself (Sarah).

I just know I was angry all the time with my children, they'd do one thing wrong that was so minor, so nothing and I'd go off [pause]... I would just scream at them, poor kids [laughs]. If they don't grow up bitter! Yeah, I'd just scream at them "what are you doing?" I wasn't a really nice person... [and] they were just scared (Lyn).

Several women like Denise and Mary had difficulty connecting with their children because of their depressive symptoms:

I was the most horrific Mum, I was like just get out of my face because I was in survival mode...she just wanted to jump on the baby and me and I said "just go away, I don't want to see you". I was just shutting off so it was pretty awful (Denise).

I know that there were days when I would lock myself in the bedroom and my four year old would have to look after the baby and the two year old. That would happen for hours at a time. I could hear the baby screaming and the toddler screaming and the older one trying to help them and being very, very good and far too much responsibility for anybody that age, but not caring... I would explain to them that I am very sad and I really need to lay down and I can't do anything for you or with you at the moment and go away basically I can't deal with you (Mary).

Attachment is a basic human need. The role of attachment is to promote a secure base for the child to grow and develop emotionally and physically. Theories of attachment and separation have been reported extensively in the literature (Ainsworth et al. 1978; Bowlby 1951, 1953, 1958, 1961, 1963, 1969; Harlow and Harlow 1962). These studies identify the importance of the bond between the mother (or caregiver) and child for the child's emotional development. The findings from our study parallel the findings from Crockenberg and Leerkes (2003) that children attach to their caregivers when they experience love and acceptance from their parents on a consistent basis. Furthermore, they found that women experienced feelings of rejection when they experienced rejection and perceived themselves as unworthy of love. Thus, the role of attachment is to promote a secure base for the child to grow and develop emotionally and physically.

The literature supports the notion that women with PND have difficulty attaching to their babies after the birth (Beck 1996; Brockington 1996; Buist 2002; Buultjens et al. 2008; Field 1998; Mauthner 2002; Mercer 1981; Ramchandani et al. 2005; O'Connor et al. 2002; Scattolon and Stoppard 1999; Sluckin 1998). The findings from our study support this claim that women with adjustment problems in pregnancy continued to have bonding problems after the birth. Buist (1996) claims that there are two groups of women with PND: those who are nurturing but have a low self-esteem and unrealistic expectations and those who have difficulty bonding with their infants and are task-oriented. Beck (1996) interviewed 12 women to explore their interactions with their infants and children when they were diagnosed with PND. Themes identified by Beck (1996) included women acting like robots when caring for their children, and at times, they erected a wall to separate themselves emotionally from their children. Similar to the findings from our study, Beck (1996) found that many women described feeling an emotional detachment from their children for months or years after the birth. Field (1998) found that depressed women have disturbed ways of communicating with their infants, such as being less affectionate and responsive to infant cues, withdrawn with flatness of affect or were hostile and intrusive. Beck and Gable (2001) showed that some women with PND detach themselves both physically and emotionally from their infants.

5.3.3   Hiding Behind a Façade of Normalcy to Preserve Self

Most women hid behind a 'façade' or 'mask' of normalcy to preserve their identities. These women applied the public mask as a means of protecting themselves from society's harsh comments and expectations and to hide their inner feelings of difficulty coping and depressive symptoms. Gammell and Stoppard (1999) reported similarly in their study of depressed women. Some women in our study found that it took too much energy to put on a facade of coping and retreated into isolation. Danni hid behind a facade of normalcy to display to others that she was coping. She described the expectations of being happy when she had her first baby:

> You just put on this pretence. You've got this new baby. "What do you mean you're not happy? Oh, isn't he beautiful?" You would put on this façade and people think that you're coping. Why wouldn't you be happy you've got a beautiful baby?

Similarly, Kristina and Tara wore a mask when they left home to hide their symptoms of depression from others:

> You put on this great mask, and you walk out the door but deep down you know it's a really dark place to be (Kristina).

> I think most people didn't know [I was depressed], I think I put up the façade. There were people who knew- close people knew that I was having a hard time (Tara).

As women perceived themselves as different to others and as failures, they hid behind a mask to hide their real or private identities and to preserve their sense of self. Therefore, their real or private identities were different to their false or public identities to create the illusion of coping. Goffman (1971) argues that these feelings generated false perceptions of what others were thinking. The preservation of the maternal identity has been reported in the literature. Maushart (1997: 21), in her book entitled, *The Mask of Motherhood*, describes the mask of motherhood as 'an assemblage of fronts, mostly brave, serene and all-knowing, that we use to disguise the chaos and complexity of our lived experience'. Charmaz (1997) argues that conflict of the dual self stems from an individual's internal dialogue – comparing self with former self and comparing self with others.

One woman in our study, Kim, felt isolated from others when she was unable to cope and imagined that others were observing her. Her sense of failure was connected to her feeling 'miserable' and unhappy, unlike other mothers who seemed to be enjoying motherhood:

> I just felt like I wasn't coping and that other people could see it. I had failed and I was failing because I wasn't happy, because I was just miserable I just didn't want them to see that I had failed that I was so miserable, I was supposed to be happy and I wasn't.

Women also hid behind a mask to give the impression of being 'good mothers'. Some women also feared their babies would be taken away if they disclosed their true feelings about motherhood. The image of the 'good mother' is commonly reported in the literature (Berggren-Clive 1998; Brown et al. 1994; Gammell and Stoppard 1999; Liamputtong 2006; Morrow et al. 2008; Nahas et al. 1999). Similar to the findings from our study, Berggren-Clive (1998) found that women set aside their own desires and wishes to attend to their children, husband and family. Furthermore, when these women put on the facade of being a 'good mother', significant people in their lives did not perceive they needed help.

Margaret, like many other participants, wanted to give the impression of being a 'good mum' as she was scared to admit that she was struggling with her own difficulties:

> You've got this thing about wanting to be a good mum [laughs]…You see everyone else around and they're all coping, so yeah I'm not going to let anyone know that I'm not.

Diane remarked:

> I think because my mother-in-law was great, she did all the cooking, at one stage she didn't even want us to do our own laundry, I just felt like I couldn't do anything. Then I started thinking, "Maybe I'm a bad mother".

Researchers have illustrated that women feared the label of the 'bad mother'. Berggren-Clive (1998) found that women with PND struggled to put a name to their experience and feared they were 'bad mothers'. Similarly, Nahas and colleagues (1999) argued that women with PND experience a fear of failure and fear of being labelled a 'bad mother' if they sought help for their depressive symptoms. Beyond Blue (2006) also found that women feared they would be ridiculed or labelled as 'bad mothers' if they disclosed their feelings. Similar to the findings from our study, Beck (1992) claimed that women perceived they were horrible mothers and failures. Also, women's obsessive thoughts of being bad mothers consumed their waking hours and isolated them from others. Rubin (1967a) suggests that women form an ideal image of themselves as mothers; this image emerges from women's perceptions of the desirable traits and achievements for maternal behaviour.

5.4   Maternal Sleep Deprivation and Emotional Well-Being

Most women described their children as 'difficult' or 'hard' and struggled with ongoing sleep deprivation. Maternal sleep deprivation is a common occurrence in the first year after the birth (Dennis and Ross 2005; Fisher and Rowe 2003). Most couples perceived that maternal sleep deprivation was a major trigger for PND, rather than being a symptom of PND. It was the chronic nature of sleep deprivation due to unsettled infant behaviour that resulted in severe fatigue and exhaustion. In their study, Buultjens and Liamputtong (2007) also found that most women with PND perceived their babies to be unsettled, and many described their babies as 'difficult', which they contributed to both sleep deprivation and to the onset of their depression.

Maternal sleep deprivation was associated with other losses – the loss of sleep, the loss of relationship (with partners and others), the loss of physical energy, the loss of control and the loss of the ability to function. Maternal sleep deprivation was also unrelated to parity as second- and third-time mothers openly discussed about being sleep-deprived because of difficulties with infant crying, sleeping and feeding. Maternal sleep deprivation was not an arbitrary amount of sleep loss but rather a chronic condition impacting on women's emotional and physical well-being in the postpartum period.

There are very few studies that have identified the impact of sleep deprivation on women's emotional well-being (Lee 1998). In the sociological literature, maternal sleep deprivation has been identified as a major contributing factor in the development of PND (Better Sleep Council 2006; Carson and Arnold 1996; Ding 2006). The Better Sleep Council (2006) found that individuals who were sleep deprived were more likely to experience depression as the lack of sleep reduces the levels of neurotransmitters in the brain, such as serotonin and dopamine. Carson and Arnold (1996) contend that sleep deprivation causes changes in the electrical activity of the brain, thereby making an individual susceptible to major depression. Furthermore, these electrical changes in the brain occur as a result of insufficient rapid eye movement (REM) sleep and are detected by electroencephalogram (EEG) (Carson and Arnold 1996).

Hunter et al. (2009) conducted a critical review of the literature to identify the nature of sleep for postpartum women and its implications for health care providers. They found that postpartum women experienced disturbances in their sleep patterns related to newborn sleep and feeding patterns. Hunter et al. (2009) concluded that providers should encourage prenatal education that aims to decrease sleep deprivation in the postnatal period.

5.4.1 Severe Fatigue/Exhaustion

Fatigue can occur when individuals get less than 6 hours of sleep in a 24 hours period (Dennis and Ross 2005), which is common with motherhood. In our study, the chronic sleep deprivation that most women experienced resulted in severe fatigue and exhaustion, and this occurred before the onset of PND. Similar to the findings of MacArthur et al. (1991), women were able to differentiate clearly between sleep deprivation and depression. As previously discussed, women in our study perceived their sleep deprivation as due to unsettled infant behaviour. These findings differ to those reported in the medical literature as most of these studies argue that PND is a cause of infant and child sleep difficulties.

In our study, women stated that they were sleep-deprived from 6 weeks to 3 years and, during that time, were socially disconnected from others as their main focus was to get the baby to sleep at all costs. The chronic nature of sleep deprivation affected women's emotional well-being and their image of themselves as mothers. Of interest, only one of these sleep-deprived mothers was bottle-feeding her infant. Breastfeeding mothers were feeding their babies frequently day and night (every 1–2 hours) leaving women with little opportunity to sleep. These findings are supported by Alder (1994) who asserted that women who breastfeed are more likely to experience fatigue than women who bottle-feed.

Women did not have the opportunity to get adequate rest or sleep to cope with motherhood as they were the primary caregivers for their infants. The partners were often working long hours and therefore unavailable to offer practical help or suggestions. Also, women felt primarily responsible for settling their infants at night to enable their partners to get some sleep. In their study, Rogan and others (1997) argued that the lack of support from others exacerbated women's feelings of fatigue. Beatrice reflected on her experience of 'fracturing' when she was unable to sleep more than an hour at a time when her baby was unsettled:

> I think when she [baby] was only six weeks old she really wasn't sleeping for more than an hour at a time and that went on for weeks and weeks and I was absolutely fracturing.

Lyn remarked that:

> I had no [emphasised] sleep [pause] but your body lives on no sleep, and then you're sleep-deprived. Then you just get to sleep and you've got a crying child, and a husband that goes off to work and thinks everything's fine. Then you're at home and think oh my God.

Samantha similarly elaborated:

> Day and night she [baby] was screaming. She didn't sleep much during the day but at night she didn't sleep much either. I felt again I was putting it on myself the pressure not to wake the others... I didn't want to wake everyone else up. [I would] rush downstairs with her so I know that was a huge thing and that went on for months.

Georgia, like most women in our study, discussed the physical effects of fatigue as a result of chronic sleep deprivation. She was exhausted and felt like she was 'going to slip into a coma' as a result of the fatigue she was experiencing. Georgia discussed the need for respite when she had reached this point:

> I was so [emphasised] exhausted most of the time, and trying to cope with that… I was really, really, really tired, you'd just start to close your eyes…it was almost feeling like you were going to slip into a coma, that tiredness… I felt like my head was going to break in half if someone didn't stop that noise…When you're really, really tired things can just [be amplified]- my skin gets sore, or I can smell things really acutely, my body hurts- there are those physical symptoms of tiredness. And noise, I stopped listening to music. I couldn't stand to hear any more noise.

Partners were also struggling with severe fatigue and had difficulty performing at work because of sleep deprivation. Brian discussed the impact of sleep deprivation on his work performance and his relationship with his wife Nancy:

> You're in a situation where you're both not sleeping… and you're not functioning properly at all levels. Everything is amplified… everything becomes more annoying- little traits in your partner that don't bother you at all become incredibly annoying.

Fatigue is more severe than tiredness which is a temporary state (McQueen and Mander 2003) and affects an individual's ability to function (Ream and Richardson 1997). McQueen and Mander (2003) found that fatigue affects an individual's physical and emotional state and can cause depression (Rogan et al. 1997; Thome and Alder 1999). McQueen and Mander (2003) suggested that severe fatigue occurred when it was chronic and not improved by rest or sleep. Rogan and associates (1997) used the category 'drained' to describe the fatigue associated with the lack of sleep and constant demands of motherhood. Researchers have argued that severe fatigue is common as a result of unsettled infant behaviour (Dennis and Ross 2005; Fisher et al. 2002). Dennis and Ross (2005) contended that the onset of depressive symptoms in the first 8 weeks postpartum is strongly associated with infant sleep patterns, maternal fatigue and sleep deprivation. They discussed the importance of night time sleep to improve maternal emotional well-being. Along a similar vein, Pugh and Milligan (1993) found that support can alleviate tiredness and fatigue in the postnatal period. Researchers have also revealed that partners experience fatigue in the postpartum period (Gay et al. 2004), but many of the studies lack the partners' perspectives. Therefore, strategies need to focus on improving the quality of sleep for both partners, with the aim of improving their emotional well-being.

5.4.2 The Unsettled Baby

When most women were unable to console their unsettled babies, they perceived they had failed as mothers. Maria expected her second baby to be more settled than her first child. She reflected back on her experience:

> Everyone said it was going to be different [that] I wouldn't have another baby that didn't sleep, and because I tried so hard to make sure that didn't happen, when it happened it was tremendously disappointing. I felt like a bit of a failure.

Elisabeth suffered from sleep deprivation for 3 years. She discussed the difficulty bonding with her daughter because of her unsettled behaviour:

> She was a really difficult baby… She was screaming day and night, the only time I could get some sleep or she could get some sleep was if she was on top of me. Beth was probably not as easy to bond with because she was such a poor sleeper and wanted to be held all the time. Every time I went to put her down she'd scream within thirty seconds, so maybe not so much [bonding] with her, even though she's easy now. She was just really difficult- she didn't start sleeping properly until she was about three.

Kath discussed the feeding problems contributing to the baby's unsettled behaviour:

> With Caitlin- it was hard to bond with her, she was a screamer you know. The midwives would walk in and go "oh, okay" [laughs], and run away as quickly as possible. I couldn't get her to breastfeed successfully… she wouldn't attach. She would suck for five seconds and then pull off, and then just start screaming so then she would get hungry, and just have this screaming cycle, and she just wouldn't settle. As soon as we got home I just expressed and bottle-fed her, and she was perfect, but they wouldn't let me try that in hospital they were adamant to breasfeed. And I thought I can't have a screaming baby, and a two year old running around being manic (Kath).

Ursula and Nicky's babies had physical problems that caused settling problems:

> [My son] had really bad reflux, His screaming used to set me off more than anything- just crying and screaming, and because it was so constant it was always ringing in my ears. And even when it wasn't him, hearing another baby would set me off… I just couldn't handle that screaming anymore. It goes straight through you. A huge amount of my day was him screaming because he was always in pain, and you know it's not his fault, and you know it's because he's in pain [and] sometimes is it that or are you just being stubborn this time? It's just too hard, and once you've heard screaming all day, for four months or whatever, you're just over it. That was my biggest trigger [for PND] (Ursula).

> The Paediatrician said, "oh, he's just a cranky little fellow!", and sort of brushed it off. And then I took him to another Paediatrician when he was ten weeks [old], and he couldn't believe that Reid- he did a pooh while I was there- and it was classic lactose intolerance. Once we took him off the breast milk and the cow's [milk] formula and put him on soy milk he was great (Nicky).

Most women with unsettled babies felt isolated from other mothers as they feared they would be judged for having an unsettled baby. The isolation from others meant that women had difficulty accessing the support they needed for validation of competence from other mothers. McQueen and Mander (2003) also found that maternal sleep deprivation affected social interaction. Ellie felt different to other mothers in the new mothers' group when her baby was unsettled:

> I remember going to mother's group, and everyone would have babies that would just sleep the whole time… [My baby] would just scream, she was just really unsettled the whole time.

Other studies echo the findings of our study. Beck (1996) identified that infant temperament was a major risk factor for PND. Pugh and Milligan (1993) argued that women who perceived their infants as difficult were more likely to experience fatigue. Tarkka (2003) found a link between maternal perceptions of children as difficult or demanding, social isolation and feelings of incompetence. In her study, the mother's ease of caring for her child affected maternal competence. In an Australian study conducted by Buultjens and Liamputtong (2007), many women with PND reported their babies as 'difficult'. Along a similar vein, Seeley et al. (1996) claimed that women with PND reported more difficulties with their infants' feeding, crying and sleeping than women without PND.

Not surprisingly, researchers have shown that when infants' sleeping patterns improve, maternal depression decreases (Armstrong et al. 1998). Some researchers have argued that women diagnosed with PND could actually be sleep-deprived and not depressed (Armstrong et al. 1998; Dennis and Ross 2005; Fisher et al. 2002; McMahon et al. 2001). In an Australian longitudinal study, McMahon and others (2001) screened 128 first-time mothers for PND when they were admitted to an early parenting centre (parent craft hospital) in New South Wales. Of these women, 73% were admitted to the early parenting centre because their babies were unsettled, and the mean age of their babies was 11 weeks. Of importance, 63% of these women met DSM-IV criteria for a major depressive episode. McMahon et al. (2001) concluded that diagnosing women with PND would not be beneficial as their episode of depression could be brief or depressive symptoms may be directly related to sleep deprivation. In a quantitative study by Dennis and Ross (2005) of 505 women, higher EPDS scores were reported at 4 and 8 weeks postpartum when women were woken at least three times overnight by their babies. Fisher and colleagues (2002) claimed that women admitted to mother-baby units with psychological distress may be inaccurately diagnosed with depression rather than fatigue related to unsettled infant behaviour.

The ongoing fatigue that women experienced resulted in the loss of control, and in some cases contributed to thoughts of hurting themselves or their infants.

5.4.3   Loss of Control

The loss of control is a common theme reported in studies of women with PND (see Berggren-Clive 1998). This theme has not been reported in studies of maternal adjustment without depressive symptoms. Most women in our study experienced the loss of control from the ongoing sleep deprivation and fatigue and had thoughts of hurting or killing themselves or their children. The loss of control was the point where women sought help for their depression and was connected to feelings of despair, helplessness and hopelessness. The feeling of losing control has been reported in studies of women with PND. Beck (1993) found that women with PND lost control of their emotions, thoughts and actions. Berggren-Clive (1998) claimed that women with PND lost control when they had thoughts of hurting themselves or their infants. In our study, the loss of control was the final stage that women experienced before they spiralled downwards into PND. Danni, a single mother, lost control when she threw her 8-month-old baby at the wall. She gave a chilling account of her experience with sleep deprivation:

> The reason that I asked for help was he had been really unsettled for quite a few weeks. I think he had been crying for about three days and I snapped one day and I just hurled him at the wall and watched him slide down it. When he hit the bed and I realised what I'd done, the look of fear in his eyes... he was eight months old. The look of fear in his eyes was just terrible.

Women also experienced the loss of control when they felt it was their responsibility to get up to their infants at night to enable their partners to get some sleep. Kath thought it was her job to get up to her children at night. The ongoing sleep deprivation resulted in the loss of control and thoughts of hurting her children. Faced with settling the children night and day, Kate lost control when she had thoughts of throwing her daughter 'through the wall':

> I feel it's my job to get up to the kids at night time... [My son] hadn't been sleeping well, neither was [my daughter]...she was having one of her hissy fits [tantrums] and [he] was bouncing off the walls driving me crazy, and I just felt that I wanted to pick her up and throw her through the wall, and that everyone would be better [off] without me because I wasn't doing a good job.

Women also experienced irrational thoughts when they lost control. Monica discussed the desperation she felt trying to get her son to sleep, and the irrational thoughts she experienced when she thought that bumping her son's head could actually help put him to sleep:

> I actually got to the point where I thought, "I nearly bumped his head there", and I thought "Oh, he might be quiet if I bump his head". And I can say it quite calmly now, and know that I would never, ever have would have intentionally hurt him but I know that went through my head... Everything was driven to just stop him from crying. That was the only time...not that I would hurt him, but if I bumped his head he might actually go to sleep for a while.

The loss of control also meant that women became angry and resentful towards their infants for not allowing them to sleep. Underneath this anger and resentment were feelings of inadequacy and incompetence for being unable to settle their infants. Georgia and Bridget commented:

> I felt like going in and shaking him. I just felt like going in and telling him how angry I was, and why wouldn't he let me sleep? And why was he doing this to me?... It didn't matter where I went in the house- there was nowhere where I seemed to be able to go where I couldn't hear this baby crying. And I just thought, I'd be better off killing myself. I could just go out now and kill myself, and that way I wouldn't feel like this, and that way I wouldn't feel like going and shaking that baby. It would be better if I went and killed myself, rather than inflicting this on my baby (Georgia).

> You do have sort of a rage inside you, like you go to put her to bed and think will you for once just go to sleep. I mean I never hurt her. The rage and control you have to have in yourself for say ten minutes while you're dealing with it, you walk outside and still know she's crying before you go back in and say "oh, alright"... I could see how some people could just get tipped over the edge and I'm sure if I just took back that time like you see on the TV what people do, you think I'm sure if I have that ten minutes over again, you could just really see how easily it could happen (Bridget).

The loss of control was also a point where most women sought help from health professionals, as Ellie and Melissa commented:

> As soon as I felt like I'd lost control I wasn't able to handle Nicky in terms of settling her [and] not feeding well, it just spiralled out of control... I remember picking Nicky [baby] up out of bed one day, and looking at her, "What do you want? I've fed you. I've burped you. You're warm- you've got enough clothes on you know. You're dry. I don't know what else to do. What do you want me to do?" I remember picking her up in a really firm, half aggressive manner, and putting her on my shoulder and you know patting her really firmly

[patting while talking]. And I just thought, "This isn't right". I put her back in the bed and I just left her and I thought, "Have a good hard look at yourself. What's going on?" It was probably at that point that I thought, "This isn't me" (Ellie).

I wanted to hurt the boys… it got to the point where I had my hands around their throats, and things like that, and I didn't hurt them but it scared Tyler quite a bit because he was old enough to sort of think, "Why has mummy got her hands around my throat. Why is she looking at me like that?" or something. I don't know, but I wanted to hurt them. I mean every parent sometimes says, "I just could kill them", but there's a difference between wanting to kill your kids and wanting to kill [emphasised] your kids. And that really scared me, because I felt like I was really out of control, and I couldn't control that, so that's what sent me to the doctor (Melissa).

The loss of control has not been reported in studies investigating the 'normal' adjustment to motherhood. However, the loss of control for women with PND has been reported in previous studies (Beck 1992, 1993, 1996; Berggren-Clive 1998; McIntosh 1993; Morgan et al. 1997; Wood et al. 1997). In the United States, Beck (1993) interviewed 12 postpartum mothers diagnosed with PND and identified the loss of control as the main psychosocial problem they encountered through the four stage process of 'Teetering on the Edge'. The stages women went through to cope with the loss of control were encountering terror, dying of self, struggling to survive and regaining control. Wood and colleagues (1997) examined the perceptions and experiences of 11 depressed mothers in the United Kingdom and found that women lost control when they felt inept at mothering. Wood et al. (1997: 312) stated, 'these mothers feel completely overwhelmed by the demands of their infants and feel trapped, angry and afraid. As time goes on these feelings continue to worsen and expand, sending mothers into a downward spiral of depression'. Similarly, Berggren-Clive (1998) interviewed eight women, who had recovered from PND in Canada, and claimed that women lost control when they spiralled downwards into depression and felt isolated from others, including their partners. Berggren-Clive (1998; 111) described the downward spiral as 'the process by which women begin to move beyond the adjustments associated with motherhood and are pulled into an absorbing and powerful vortex'.

5.5   Chapter Summary

For most women in the study, the adjustment to motherhood represented a time when they were faced with profound physical, emotional and social changes. Motherhood was a significant time in these women's lives, yet the reality of motherhood was vastly different to their expectations, particularly in relation to support. The majority of primiparous women and their partners described feeling unprepared for parenthood despite attending antenatal classes, meeting with health professionals, accessing internet sites and reading books.

The unmet expectations of support from partners, friends and especially their own mothers resulted in feelings of disappointment, loss of self-esteem and isolation from others. However, most women reported distant relationships with their mothers which meant they had difficulty accessing emotional support, practical help, mothering skills and reassurance for their sense of competence and self-esteem. As a result of this emotional disconnection with women's own mothers, there was the lack of practical skills of mothering passed down from mother to daughter for women to learn how to be mothers.

The loss of self was one of the most significant losses that women experienced and resulted from multiple losses, such as the loss of independence, the temporary loss of their career and the loss of work relationships. Women lost their sense of self when they felt different to other mothers, and they struggled to find their identities. They struggled to give the impression of being a 'good mother' to protect their identities by hiding behind a mask to hide their depressive symptoms and inability to cope.

Maternal sleep deprivation was not an arbitrary amount of sleep loss, but a chronic condition impacting on women's emotional and physical well-being in the postpartum period. As a result of the severe fatigue and exhaustion that women experienced, they were too tired to interact with others and wanted to settle their babies in the privacy of their own homes. The isolation from others meant that women had difficulty accessing support from others such as emotional support, reassurance or validation of maternal competences. The lack of support from health professionals about settling techniques meant that women were trying to settle their babies by themselves with no strategies to deal with their unsettled infants.

The ongoing sleep deprivation that women experienced resulted in the loss of control where they had thoughts of hurting or killing themselves or their children. The loss of control was the point most women reached where they sought help for their depression. The feeling of loss of control was connected to women being unable to settle their infants and contributed to the sense of failure that women experienced.

This chapter highlights the need for increased support in early motherhood and identifies the need for informational support and advice from health professionals. Women wanted emotional support and validation of maternal competence from other women, particularly their own mothers. They also expected their own mothers to provide practical help and advice to support them when they became mothers. This resulted in women struggling alone with little support and guidance. The following chapter will detail how women and their partners understand and explain PND. Women's drawings will add to their verbal accounts of PND to provide rich descriptions of their experiences.

References

Ainsworth, M. D. S., Blehar, M., Waters, E., & Wall, S. (1978). *Patterns of attachment*. Hillsdale: Erlbaum.
Alder, B. (1994). The psychology of mood and sex in pregnancy and the puerperium. In P. Y. L. Choi & P. Nicholson (Eds.), *pi*. New York: Harvester Wheatsheaf.
Allan, S., & Gilbert, P. (1997). Submissive behaviour and psychopathology. *The British Journal of Clinical Psychology, 36*, 467–488.

American Psychiatric Association. (2000). *Diagnostic and statistical manual of mental disorders, text revision. DSM-IV-TR (4th revised ed.).* Washington, DC: American Psychiatric Press.

Appleby, L., Warner, R., Whitton, A., & Faragher, B. (1997). A controlled study of fluoxetine and cognitive-behavioural counselling in the treatment of postnatal depression. *British Medical Journal, 314*(7085), 932–936. March.

Armstrong, K. L., Van Haeringen, A. R., Dadds, M. R., & Cash, R. (1998). Sleep deprivation or postnatal depression in later infancy: Separating the chicken from the egg. *Journal of Paediatrics and Child Health, 34*(3), 260–262.

Barclay, L., & Lloyd, B. (1996). The misery of motherhood: Alternative approaches to maternal distress. *Midwifery, 12*, 136–139.

Barclay, L. B., Everitt, L., Rogan, F., Schmied, V., & Wyllie, A. (1997). 'Becoming a mother' -an analysis of women's experience of early motherhood. *Journal of Advanced Nursing, 25*, 719–728.

Barlow, C., & Cairns, K. (1997). Mothering as a psychological experience. *Canadian Journal of Counseling, 31*(3), 232–237.

Beck, C. T., (1992). The lived experience of postpartum depression: A phenomenological study. *Nursing Research, 41*(3), 166–170.

Beck, C. T., (1993). Teetering on the edge: A substantive theory of postpartum depression. *Nursing Research, 42*, 42–48.

Beck, C. T., (1996). Postpartum depressed mothers' experiences interacting with their children. *Nursing Research, 45*, 98–104.

Beck, C. T., (1999). Postpartum depression: Stopping the thief that steals motherhood. *AWHONN Lifelines, 3*(4), 41–44.

Beck, C. T., (2002). Postnatal depression: A metasynthesis. *Qualitative Health Research, 12*(4), 453–472.

Beck, C. T., & Gable, R. K. (2001). Further validation of the postpartum depression screening scale. *Nursing Research, 50*(3), 155–164.

Beck, C. T., & Indman, P. (2005). The many faces of postpartum depression. *Journal of Obstetric, Gynecologic, and Neonatal Nursing, 34*(5), 569–576.

Berggren-Clive, K. (1998). Out of the darkness and into the light: Women's experiences with depression of childbirth. *Canadian Journal of Community Mental Health, 17*, 103–120.

Bergum, V. (1986). *The phenomenology from woman to mother.* Unpublished doctoral dissertation. Alberta: University of Alberta

Better Sleep Council. (2006). The critical link between sleep and emotional well-being. http://www.bettersleep.org/emotional-well-being.asp. Accessed 8 Aug 2006.

Beyond Blue. (2006). What is postnatal depression? http://www.beyondblue.org.au/index. aspx?link_id=94. Accessed 12 June 2007.

Birchwood, M., Meaden, A., Trower, P., Gilbert, P., & Plaistow, J. (2000). The power and omnipotence of voices: Subordination and entrapment by voices and significant others. *Psychological Medicine, 30*, 337–344.

Bowlby, J. (1951). *Maternal care and mental health.* New York: Sckocken.

Bowlby, J. (1953). Some pathological processes set in train by early mother-child separation. *The Journal of Mental Science, 99*, 265–272.

Bowlby, J. (1958). The nature of the child's tie to his mother. *International Journal of Psycho-Analysis, 39*, 350–373.

Bowlby, J. (1961). Separation anxiety: A critical review of the literature. *Journal of Child Psychology and Psychiatry, 1*, 251–269.

Bowlby, J. (1963). Pathological mourning and childhood mourning. *Journal of American Psychoanalytic Association, 11*, 500–541.

Bowlby, J. (1969). *Attachment and loss* (Vol. 1). New York: Basic Books.

Brockington, I. (1996). *Motherhood and mental health.* Oxford: Oxford University Press.

Bromwich, R. M. (1976). Focus on maternal behavior in infant intervention. *The American Journal of Orthopsychiatry, 46*, 439–446.

Brown, G. W. (1998). Genetic and population perspectives on life events and depression. *Social Psychiatry and Psychiatric Epidemiology, 33*, 363–372.

Brown, G. W., Bifulco, A., & Harris, T. O. (1987). Life events, vulnerability and onset of depression: Some refinements. *The British Journal of Psychiatry, 150*, 30–42.

Brown, S., Lumley, J., Small, R., & Astbury, J. (1994). *Missing voices. The experience of motherhood*. Melbourne: Oxford University Press.

Brown, G. W., Harris, T. O., & Hepworth, C. (1995). Loss, humiliation and entrapment among women developing depression: A patient and non-patient comparison. *Psychological Medicine, 25*(1), 7–22.

Brown, S., Small, R., Faber, B., Krastev, A., & Davis, P. (2003). Early postnatal discharge from hospital for healthy mothers and term infants. *Cochrane Database for Systematic Reviews, 1*, No page number.

Buist, A. (1996). *Psychiatric disorders associated with childbirth*. Sydney: McGraw-Hill.

Buist, A. (2002). Mental health in pregnancy: The sleeping giant. *Australasian Psychiatry, 10*(3), 203–206.

Busfield, J. (1996). *Men, women and madness. Understanding gender and mental disorder*. London: MacMillan.

Buultjens, M., & Liamputtong, P. (2007). When giving life starts to take the life out of you: Women's experiences of depression after childbirth. *Midwifery, 23*, 77–91.

Buultjens, M., Robinson, P., & Liamputtong, P. (2008). A holistic programme for mothers with postnatal depression: Pilot study. *Journal of Advanced Nursing, 63*(2), 181–188.

Carson, V. B., & Arnold, E. N. (1996). *Mental health nursing. The nurse-patient journey*. Philadelphia: W.B. Saunders.

Chaffin, M., Kelleher, K., & Hollenberg, J. (1996). Onset of physical abuse and neglect: Psychiatric, substance abuse, and social risk factors from prospective community data. *Child Abuse & Neglect, 20*(3), 191–203.

Charmaz, K. (1997). Identity dilemmas of chronically ill men. In A. Strauss & J. Corbin (Eds.), *Grounded theory in practice*. Thousand Oaks: Sage.

Costello, C. (1976). *Anxiety and depression*. Montreal: McGill-Queen's University Press.

Crockenberg, S. C., & Leerkes, E. M. (2003). Parental acceptance, postpartum depression, and maternal sensitivity: Mediating and moderating processes. *Journal of Family Psychology, 17*(1), 80–93.

Crouch, M., & Manderson, L. (1993). *New motherhood. Cultural and personal transitions*. Melbourne: Gordon and Breach.

Dalton, K. (1996). *Depression after childbirth* (3rd ed.). Oxford: Oxford University Press.

Dennis, C. L., & Ross, L. (2005). Relationships among infant sleep patterns, maternal fatigue, and development of depressive symptomatology. *Birth, 32*(3), 187–193.

Ding, K. (2006). New parenthood and sleep deprivation. http://www.ahealthyme.com/topic/sleepdeprive. Accessed 12 June 2007.

Dix, C. (1987). *The new mother syndrome. Coping with post-natal stress and depression*. Sydney: Allen & Unwin.

Driscoll, J. W. (1990). Maternal parenthood and the grief process. *The Journal of Perinatal and Neonatal Nursing, 4*(2), 1–10.

Eriksen, K., & Kress, V. E. (2005). *Beyond the DSM story*. Thousand Oaks: Sage.

Field, T. (1998). Maternal depression effects on infants and early interventions. *Preventative Medicine, 27*(27), 200–203.

Fisher, J. F., & Rowe, H. J. (2003). *Building an evidence base for practice in early parenting centres. A systematic review of the literature and a report of an outcome study*. Melbourne: Tweddle Child and Family Health Services.

Fisher, J. R. W., Feekery, C. J., & Rowe-Murray, H. J. (2002). Nature, severity and correlates of psychological distress in women admitted to a private mother-baby unit. *Journal of Paediatrics and Child Health, 38*(2), 140.

Fowles, E. R. (1998). The relationship between maternal role attainment and postpartum depression. *Health Care for Women International, 19*, 83–94.

Gammell, D. J., & Stoppard, J. M. (1999). Women's experiences of treatment of depression: Medicalization or empowerment? *Canadian Psychology, 40*(2), 112–128.

Gay, C. L., Lee, K. A., & Lee, S. Y. (2004). Sleep patterns and fatigue in new mothers and fathers. *Biological Research for Nursing, 5*(4), 311–318.

Gilbert, P., & Allan, S. (1998). The role of defeat and entrapment (arrested flight) in depression: An exploration of an evolutionary view. *Psychological Medicine, 28*(3), 585–598.

Gjerdingen, D., Froberg, D., & Fontaine, P. (1991). The effects of social support on women's health during pregnancy, labor and delivery, and the postpartum period. *Family Medicine, 23*, 370–375.

Goffman, E. (1961). *Asylums*. Hammondsworth: Penguin.

Goffman, E. (1963). *Stigma: Notes on the management of spoiled identity*. Ringwood: Penguin Books.

Goffman, E. (1971). *Relations in public: Microstudies of the public order*. New York: Basic Books.

Goffman, E. (1972). *Interaction ritual. Essays on face-to-face behaviour*. London: Allen Lane The Penguin Press.

Gottlieb, L. N., & Mendelson, M. J. (1995). Mothers' moods and social support when a second child is born. *Maternal-Child Nursing Journal, 23*(1), 3–14.

Gramling, S. E., & Auerbach, S. (2006). *Stress (psychology) Microsoft Encarta Online Encyclopedia*. http://www.encarta.msn.com/text_761572052__0/Stress_(psychology).html. Accessed 23 May 2006.

Harlow, H., & Harlow, M. (1962). Social deprivation in monkeys. *Scientific American, 207*(5), 136.

Hart, M. M. (1981). Becoming a mother: Motherhood from the woman's perspective (Doctoral dissertation, Pennsylvania State University). *Dissertation Abstracts International, 42*(4B), 1633–1634.

Holopainen, D. (2002). The experience of seeking help for postnatal depression. *Journal of Advanced Nursing, 19*(3), 39–44.

Hunter, L. P., Rychnovsky, J. D., & Yount, S. M. (2009). A selective review of maternal sleep characteristics in the postpartum period. *Journal of Obstetric, Gynecologic, and Neonatal Nursing, 38*, 6–68.

Hurst, S. A. (1999). Legacy of betrayal: A grounded theory of becoming demoralized from the perspective of women who have been depressed. *Canadian Psychology, 40*(2), 179–191.

Kauffman, M. (2003). Appearances, stigma, and prevention. *Remedial and Special Education, 24*(4), 195 (194).

Keating-Lefler, R., & Wilson, M. E. (2004). The experience of becoming a mother for single, unpartnered, medicaid-eligible, first-time mothers. *Journal of Nursing Scholarship, 36*(1), 23–29.

Kiehl, E. M., & White, M. A. (2003). Maternal adaptation during childbearing in Norway, Sweden, and the United States. *Scandinavian Journal of Caring Sciences, 17*, 96–103.

Kitzinger, S. (1992). *Ourselves as mothers. The universal experience of motherhood*. London: Doubleday.

Kivijarvi, M., Raiha, H., Virtanen, S., Lertola, K., & Piha, J. (2004). Maternal sensitivity behaviour and infant crying, fussing and contented behaviour: The effects of mother's experienced social support. *Scandinavian Journal of Psychology, 45*, 239–246.

Lauer-Williams, J. (2001). Postpartum depression: A phenomenological exploration of the woman's experience. *Dissertation Abstracts International: Section B: The Sciences & Engineering, 62*(4-B), 2064.

Lee, K. A. (1998). Alterations in sleep during pregnancy and postpartum: A review of 30 years of research. *Sleep Medicine Reviews, 2*(4), 231–242.

Leff, J., Vearnals, S., & Brewin, C. R. (2000). The London Depression Intervention Trial: Randomised controlled trial of antidepressants v. Couple therapy in the treatment and maintenance of people with depression living with a partner: Clinical outcome and costs. *The British Journal of Psychiatry, 177*, 95–100.

Liamputtong, P. (2006). Motherhood and "moral career": Discourses of good motherhood among Southeast Asian immigrant women in Australia. *Qualitative Sociology, 29*(1), 25–53.

Liamputtong, P. (2007). *The journey of becoming a mother amongst women in northern Thailand.* Lanham: Lexington Books.

Liamputtong, P., & Naksook, C. (2003). Life as mothers in a new land: The experience of motherhood among Thai women in Australia. *Health Care for Women International, 24,* 650–668.

MacArthur, C., Lewis, M., & Knox, E. G. (1991). *Health after childbirth.* London: HMSO.

Martins, C., & Gaffan, E. A. (2000). Effects of early maternal depression on patterns of infant-mother attachment: A meta-analytic investigation. *Journal of Child Psychology and Psychiatry, 41,* 737–746.

Maushart, S. (1997). *The mask of motherhood.* Sydney: Random House.

Mauthner, N. S. (1995). Postnatal depression: The significance of social contacts between mothers. *Women's Studies International Forum, 18,* 311–323.

Mauthner, N. S. (1999). "Feeling low and feeling really bad about feeling low": Women's experiences of motherhood and postpartum depression. *Canadian Psychology, 40*(2), 143–161.

Mauthner, N. S. (2002). *The darkest days of my life. Stories of postpartum depression.* Cambridge: Harvard University Press.

McIntosh, J. (1993). Postpartum depression: Women's help-seeking behaviour and perceptions of cause. *Journal of Advanced Nursing, 18,* 178–184.

McMahon, M. (1995). *Engendering motherhood: Identity and self-transformation in women's lives.* New York: The Guilford Press.

McMahon, C., Barnett, B., Kowalenko, N., Tennant, C., & Don, N. (2001). Postnatal depression, anxiety and unsettled infant behaviour. *The Australian and New Zealand Journal of Psychiatry, 35*(5), 581.

McQueen, A., & Mander, R. (2003). Tiredness and fatigue in the postnatal period. *Journal of Advanced Nursing, 42*(5), 463–469.

McVeigh, C. (1997). Motherhood experiences from the perspective of first-time mothers. *Clinical Nursing Research, 6*(4), 335–348.

Mead, G. (1934). *Mind, self and society.* Chicago: University of Chicago Press.

Mercer, R. T. (1981). A theoretical framework for studying factors that impact on the maternal role. *Nursing Research, 30,* 73–77.

Mercer, R. T. (1985). The process of maternal role attainment over the first year. *Nursing Research, 34,* 198–204.

Mercer, R. T. (2004). Becoming a mother versus maternal role attainment. *Journal of Nursing Scholarship, 36,* 226–232.

Milgrom, J., Martin, P. R., & Negri, L. M. (1999). *Treating postnatal depression. A psychological approach for health care practitioners.* Chichester: Wiley.

Morgan, M., Matthey, S., Barnett, B., & Richardson, C. (1997). A group program for postnatally distressed women and their partners. *Journal of Advanced Nursing, 26,* 913–920.

Morrow, M., Smith, J., Lai, Y., & Jaswal, S. (2008). Shifting landscapes: Immigrant women and post partum depression. *Health Care for Women International, 29*(6), 593–617.

Nahas, V. L., & Amasheh, N. (1999). Culture care meanings and experiences of postpartum depression among Jordanian Australian women: A transcultural study. *Journal of Transcultural Nursing, 10,* 37–45.

Nahas, V. L., Hillege, S., & Amasheh, N. (1999). International exchange. Postpartum depression: The lived experiences of Middle Eastern migrant women in Australia. *Journal of Nurse-Midwifery, 44*(1), 65–74.

Nelson, A. M. (2003). Transition to motherhood. *Journal of Obstetric, Gynecologic, and Neonatal Nursing, 32*(4), 465–477.

Nicolson, P. (1990). Understanding postnatal depression: A mother-centred approach. *Journal of Advanced Nursing, 15,* 689–695.

Nicolson, P. (1999). Loss, happiness and postpartum depression: The ultimate paradox. *Canadian Psychology, 40*(2), 162–178.

Nims, C. L. (1996). *Postpartum depression: The lived experience.* Unpublished Master's thesis. Toledo: Medical College of Ohio.

Nolan, M. L. (1997). Antenatal education- Where next? *Journal of Advanced Nursing, 25*(6), 1198–1204.

Oakley, A. (1980). *Women confined. Towards a sociology of childbirth.* Oxford: Martin Robinson.

O'Connor, T. G., Heron, J., & Glover, V. (2002). Antenatal anxiety predicts child behavioural/ emotional problems independently of postnatal depression. *Journal of the American Academy of Child and Adolescent Psychiatry, 41*(12), 1470–1477.

Paris, R., & Dubus, N. (2005). Staying connected while nurturing and infant: A challenge of new motherhood. *Family Relations, 54*, 72–83.

Pease, B., & Wilson, J. (1995). Men in families: Moving beyond patriarchal relations. In W. Weeks & J. Wilson (Eds.), *Issues facing Australian families. Human services respond.* Melbourne: Longman.

Podkolinski, J. (1998). Women's experience of postnatal support. In S. Clement (Ed.), *Psychological perspectives on pregnancy and childbirth.* Edinburgh: Churchill Livingstone.

Pridham, K. F., Chang, A. S., & Chiu, Y. M. (1994). Mothers' parenting self-appraisals: The contribution of perceived infant temperament. *Research in Nursing and Health, 17*, 381–392.

Pugh, L. C., & Milligan, R. M. (1993). A framework for the study of childbearing fatigue. *Advances in Nursing Science, 15*, 60–70.

Putnam, R. D. (2000). *Bowling alone. The collapse and revival of American community.* New York: Simon & Schuster.

Ramchandani, P., Stein, A., Evans, J., & O'Connor, T. G. (2005). Paternal depression in the postnatal period and child development: A prospective population study. *Lancet, 365*, 2201–2205.

Ream, E., & Richardson, A. (1997). Fatigue: A concept analysis. *International Journal of Nursing Studies, 33*, 519–529.

Rogan, F., Shmied, V., Barclay, L., Everett, L., & Wyllie, A. (1997). 'Becoming a mother'-developing a new theory of early motherhood. *Journal of Advanced Nursing, 25*, 877–885.

Rubin, R. (1961). Basic maternal behaviour. *Nursing Outlook, 9*, 683–686.

Rubin, R. (1967). Attainment of the maternal role. Part 1. Processes. *Nursing Research, 16*, 237–245.

Rubin, R. (1984). *Maternal identity and the maternal experience.* New York: Springer.

Scattolon, W., & Stoppard, J. M. (1999). "Getting on with life": Women's experiences and ways of coping with depression. *Canadian Psychology, 40*(2), 205–219.

Seeley, S., Murray, L., & Cooper, P. J. (1996). The outcome for mothers and babies of health visitor intervention. *Health Visitor, 69*, 135–138.

Semprevivo, D. M. (1996). *The lived experience of postpartum mental illness.* Thousand Oaks: Sage.

Sluckin, A. (1998). Bonding failure: 'I don't know this baby, she's nothing to do with me'. *Clinical Child Psychology and Psychiatry, 3*(1), 11–24.

Smith, M. (2002). Stigma. *Advances in psychiatric treatment, 8*, 317–325.

Tammentie, T., Paavilainen, E., Astedt-Kurki, P., & Tarkka, M.-T. (2004). Family dynamics of postnatally depressed mothers- discrepancy between expectations and reality. *Journal of Clinical Nursing, 13*(1), 65–74.

Tarkka, M.-T. (2003). Predictors of maternal competence by first-time mothers when the child is 8 months old. *Journal of Advanced Nursing, 41*(3), 233–240.

Thome, M., & Alder, B. (1999). A telephone intervention to reduce fatigue and symptom distress in mothers with difficult infants in the community. *Journal of Advanced Nursing, 29*, 128–137.

Thompson, V. L. S., Noel, J. G., & Campbell, J. (2004). Stigmatization, discrimination, and mental health: The impact of multiple identity status. *The American Journal of Orthopsychiatry, 74*(4), 529–544.

Tomison, A. M. (1996). Child maltreatment and mental disorder. *Discussion Paper Number 3*, 1–19.
Underdown, A. (1998). Parenthood: The transition to parenthood. *British Journal of Midwifery*, *6*(8), 508–511.
WHO. (1999). Postpartum care of the mother and newborn: A practical guide. *Birth, 26*(4), 255–258.
Wilkinson, R. B., & Mulcahy, R. (2010). Attachment and interpersonal relationships in postnatal depression. *Journal of Reproductive and Infant Psychology, 28*(3), 252–265.
Wood, A. F., Thomas, S. P., Droppleman, P. G., & Meighan, M. (1997). The downward spiral of postpartum depression. *Maternal-Child Nursing Journal, 22*, 308–317.

Chapter 6
'Postnatal': Trapped, Alone in the Dark – Women's Experiences of Postnatal Depression and Drawings

> I remember the time as if I was in a permanent fog. I went through the motions every day but felt numb a lot of the time. I felt hopeless and useless that I was not coping and could not admit that I wasn't. I felt lonely, isolated and guilty that I was not appreciating the wonderful little baby I just had (Sarah).

Most women in this study, like Sarah, felt isolated and alone when they were depressed, even though all but one of the women was partnered when they were diagnosed with PND. Sarah's quote highlights the sense of isolation and hopelessness the women who were diagnosed with PND experienced. In this chapter, we will explore couples' experiences of screening and diagnosis of PND and their perceptions of the label of PND. " 'Postnatal', Trapped alone in the dark" represents the darkness, isolation and feeling of entrapment that most women experienced when they developed PND. The couples used the term 'postnatal' when they talked about PND, perhaps to avoid labelling their experiences as PND. 'Postnatal' may refer to a period of distress rather than depression in motherhood.

The women's drawings depicted in this chapter provide powerful visual images of their lived experience of PND and enhance their verbal accounts. In this chapter, we also detail the amount of support partners provided to women, as well as the couples' perceptions of their relationship, and the emotional health of the partners. When women developed PND, they need support from their partners when they develop depressive symptoms, as many partners assisted women to treatment.

6.1 The Process of Diagnosis

Most women experienced one episode of PND (range of one to three episodes). What was evident from their stories was the range of biopsychosocial factors that contributed to depressive symptoms, particularly social factors. Only a small number

C. Westall and P. Liamputtong, *Motherhood and Postnatal Depression: Narratives of Women and Their Partners*, DOI 10.1007/978-94-007-1694-0_6,
© Springer Science+Business Media B.V. 2011

of women developed symptoms of PND within 4 weeks of childbirth. The latest onset of PND reported was 10 months after birth. These findings are congruent with the findings in literature that symptoms of PND occur within 12 months of childbirth (Brown et al. 1994; Milgrom et al. 1999; Ugarriza 2002). Similar to the findings from our study, Brown and colleagues (1994) revealed that over one third of women developed symptoms of PND after 3 months of childbirth.

In our study, women were diagnosed with PND by various health professionals, such as maternal and child health nurses, general practitioners, psychologists, social workers, obstetricians, early parenting centres and mother–baby units. Only four women self-identified as having PND and these cases were confirmed by General Practitioners. These women stated: 'I pretty much diagnosed myself and that's why I went to the doctor' (Mary); 'I rang [mum] up bawling saying, 'Mum, I think I have postnatal depression. I need to go to the doctors" (Meg). This echoes findings in the literature that women who are depressed are unlikely to recognise symptoms of depression or discuss them with a health professional (Beyond Blue 2006; Whitton et al. 1996).

Only a few women were uncertain where they could access help for PND. In her study, Holopainen (2002) claimed that one woman out of seven interviewed in Melbourne did not know where to seek professional help. In our study, Kim, a first-time mother, was unaware where to access help when she was depressed. She discussed the dilemma of trying to find a counsellor when she was depressed:

> We thought about trying to get some counselling, but didn't know where to start looking…
> I wanted help. I was going to do anything to get help. One of our friends she had seen a counsellor and I'm like 'how did you find out?' She said, 'I was desperate I just went through the yellow pages'. If that hadn't worked out with the psychologist, I would have got the yellow pages out.

Although most women were aware of support services, they had difficulty asking for help. As a result, partners, family members, friends and neighbours were instrumental in convincing women they needed professional help and assessment.

6.1.1   Screening and Diagnosis

Most women were diagnosed with PND following screening with the Edinburgh Postnatal Depression Scale (EPDS). In general, women found the EPDS to be an acceptable screening tool, as comments such as 'I was happy to do it' were commonly expressed during the interviews. These findings differ from Shakespeare and colleagues (2003) who found that over half of the sample of 22, women had negative perceptions of the EPDS. The difference in these findings could possibly be due to sample differences as not all women were depressed in Shakespeare et al. (2003) study.

Some women who were screened with the EPDS were dishonest when they completed the EPDS as they perceived they were failures or bad mothers or not ready to admit they were depressed. Interestingly, these women met the criteria for PND when screened. This indicates that instead of scoring three on specific items, they would have to score one or two on most questions as they would need to have a total score of above 12 to screen positively for PND. This finding indicates that women who score above 12 could have scores higher than recorded. Women with lower scores could also be depressed. This is a particular concern for question 10 that asks about self-harm. Even when women downplayed their answers, their scores were above the cut-off score of 12, indicating probable depression. Val discussed the quandary she experienced when faced with completing the EPDS and not coping:

> Most of the time I could answer [the EPDS] quite honestly… I had done that a couple of times… I wasn't ready to admit it [PND] to me. If you're not ready to admit it to yourself you can't to others, and I was very good at hiding it, no-one knew. I knew things weren't right but…I really just wasn't prepared for saying, 'I'm not coping'.

Similarly, Margaret admitted to lying on the EPDS, as she wanted to be a 'good mum'.

> I remember sort of lying…you've got this thing about wanting to be a good mum [laughs]… You see everyone else around and they are all coping so yeah I'm not going to let anyone know that I'm not [coping].

Maria also confessed to lying when she completed the EPDS. She was concerned that her maternal and child health nurse would lock her up if she completed it honestly:

> I knew myself that I had in fact lied on the thing [EPDS]. I hadn't been honest. It [depression] was actually worse, it [the EPDS score] would have been a lot higher. She [maternal and child health nurse] would have locked me up or something. I just didn't know what she would do if she did find out it was high. I was scared of that.

Bridget was also dishonest when she completed the EPDS as she was worried about the consequences of being suicidal:

> I thought it [EPDS] was a bit vague actually…If you do answer a question…"Are you suicidal?"… 'Yes'…What is going to be the consequence of that? You wouldn't answer it honestly… because there might be consequences.

Although Sue had difficulty completing the EPDS honestly, she expressed the importance of being honest with herself so she could get help for her depressive symptoms:

> It was really hard to be truthful with myself and not try and make it look better than it is because that's your tendency, I'm really not that bad. To really be honest with myself and with the doctors so I could actually get the help was very hard because I was in denial, I didn't want to believe that I was as depressed as I was. It was very hard to fill out.

Shakespeare and colleagues (2003) also identified that women in their study were dishonest when they completed the EPDS. However, their participants wanted to avoid disappointing their health visitor by scoring honestly. Our study differed as women scored dishonestly because they were not ready to admit to themselves that they were depressed and perceived themselves as failures and 'bad mothers'. From a different standpoint, Cox and Holden (2003) stated in validation studies, where the EPDS was compared with a diagnostic interview, that most women completed the EPDS accurately. In our study, the fact that some lied on the EPDS highlights the need for a clinical interview to follow screening to explore how women are feeling and to identify the risk of self-harm or harming their children. Also, this finding indicates the need for informational support to dispel the myth of the perfect mother and to discuss the reality of motherhood.

6.1.2 The Label of 'Postnatal' Depression

Many women were ambivalent at the time of diagnosis and had difficulty accepting the label of PND as there were so many personal and social factors that impacted on their emotional well-being. This could be the reason why the majority of women and their partners used the term 'postnatal' when they discussed their experiences of PND. Perhaps couples wanted to avoid labelling their experiences as PND. 'Postnatal' may refer to a period of distress rather than depression in motherhood. What we have found has not been reported in the literature and was central to all of the interviews. The couples' use of the term 'postnatal' is interspersed throughout the chapter. A quote from a partner, Nick, in the focus group interview highlights this point:

> Do you isolate it out and say, 'That's postnatal or just underlying depression, and self-esteem issues?'

Most couples were aware that there was something wrong and that women had difficulty in coping with motherhood. However, these couples were unable to identify that women were depressed as they perceived that their situation was affecting women's emotional well-being. Similar to the findings from our study, McIntosh (1993) showed that 97% of women recognised that something was wrong, but only 32% realised that they were suffering from PND. Whitton and colleagues (1996) claimed that women knew that something was not right, but perceived that it was normal to feel miserable after birth; health visitors also held this belief. Our study adds that partners were also aware that something was wrong. Noah, like most of the partners, was aware that there was something not right with his wife as she had difficulty coping. He described the helplessness he experienced when his wife was depressed as he was unsure what to do to relieve the depressive symptoms:

> I don't know that I'd pinpoint it as PND but I knew that there was something wrong and that she wasn't coping for a long time. It was really starting to scare me because I didn't really know what to do about it.

Several women acknowledged that their personality type or psychological factors contributed to the development of their PND. These women identified themselves as 'anxious', 'perfectionists' or 'control freaks'. Brown and Harris (1978) argue that even if women have personality traits, changing their environment could lessen their risk of developing depression, for example, providing more support to women. However, most couples in our study discussed the combination of factors that contributed to PND. The majority of these factors were external rather than internal. Similar findings have been reported in the literature (Buultjens and Liamputtong 2007; McIntosh 1993; Morrow et al. 2008; Scattolon and Stoppard 1999; Ugarriza 2002). In their study, Scattolon and Stoppard (1999) contended that women felt their depression was caused by external life stressors and, to a lesser extent, by hormonal or medical reasons. One woman in our study, Elisabeth, like many women, attributed her PND due to a combination of factors. She perceived that having a difficult toddler and an unsettled baby contributed to her symptoms of PND:

> I don't think it was at the time… postnatal. I thought it was a combination of things – having a baby that wasn't sleeping as well as having a difficult toddler. I didn't realise that together that could still be classified as postnatal depression.

Most of the men also agreed that PND occurred due to a combination of factors. We were unable to locate any studies that explored the partners' explanations of PND. One partner in the focus group, Michael, mentioned the 'other things' that contributed to PND rather than just the addition of the baby:

> It's never in my opinion right the baby came along, bang, it [PND] started. It was always other things.

At the time of diagnosis, women and their partners were also confused about what PND was and had little understanding of the condition. The lack of understanding and feeling of confusion at the time of diagnosis may have been contributed to insufficient information about PND being given to couples to enable them to understand the condition. One partner, Brian, was confused about the label of PND, especially when there are individual expressions of the condition:

> You can label it as that [PND] but then again see what is it? What is it? I can see it's so varied, it's something different from minute to minute…for every single person it's a different thing, and every day it's a different thing. And different triggers, different days, and different times…it's such a varied thing.

Some of the partners were initially ambivalent about their diagnosis of PND because they rejected the label of PND. Previous research has reported similar findings. Whitton and colleagues (1996) revealed that 55% of women thought their symptoms were not severe enough to be labelled as depression. Along a similar vein, Brown and others (1994) claimed that women disagreed with the label of PND and if contributed their feelings to their workload or tiredness.

The partners were more likely to agree with the diagnosis of PND as compared with women. Most of the men agreed with their partners' diagnosis of PND. They discussed how the diagnosis of PND 'made sense', 'fell into place', was 'not really a surprise' and 'didn't disagree'. Shane was ambivalent about the diagnosis of PND:

> I didn't disagree [with the diagnosis of PND] but I've known Kelly through suffering depression anyway and I didn't know if it was postnatal or a continuation on of her depression... I know she was very disappointed with the birth process.

Women's poor understanding of PND resulted in feelings of disbelief when they were diagnosed with the condition. Most women, like Sue, were aware that the baby blues was less severe than PND. She was confused and shocked when she was diagnosed with PND:

> I had heard about the baby blues, and I had heard about postnatal depression, but postnatal depression in my mind was a severe case, people don't get that, so why would I get it? It was a big shock. I didn't know how to accept it.

Melissa also discussed how the diagnosis of PND was 'a little bit strange', as she was unaware of the condition of PND. She discussed knowing more about cancer than depression at the time of diagnosis:

> It felt a little bit strange because I just never, never really had ever discussed it or come across it or anything. If it was cancer it would have meant more to me than depression. I guess there's a bit of a stigma with depression.

6.1.3 Relief

Although women challenged the label of PND, in general, they were relieved that something could be done to improve their emotional well-being. Women reached a point where they were unable to hide behind the mask. Gammell and Stoppard (1999) and Mauthner (2002) have also reported similarly. One woman, Val, reached a point where she was unable to hide her feelings anymore. She was relieved to know that help was available to escape the misery she was experiencing:

> I think I felt relieved. It was out there then, there was no hiding the fact, I'd lost all chances of that [laughs]. And I think I had got to the stage where I needed help and I was relieved that there was someone there that could help me.

Similar feelings of relief were expressed by Monica. Although Monica was uncertain if she was depressed or had developed post-traumatic stress disorder as a result of her birth experience, she was relieved to know that there was something she could do:

> I think at the time I was relieved to have someone say to me, "There's something we can do to help". I think I pretty much knew that I was suffering from something. I think we never really drew the line between whether it was one-hundred percent postnatal depression or post-traumatic stress...but I was just relieved that there was something I could do.

Studies have found that some women are relieved when they are diagnosed with PND (Mauthner 2002), while others reported women feeling stigmatised and labelled by the condition (Brockington 1996; Gammell and Stoppard 1999; Scattolon and Stoppard 1999). Although some women in our study were relieved by the medical diagnosis of PND, others were concerned about the stigma of being labelled with a form of mental illness.

6.1.4   Stigma

The stigma of mental illness meant that the women perceived themselves to be less competent than other mothers, and this added to the sense of failure they were already experiencing. The stigma that the women experienced was evident when they used the following metaphors to describe themselves: 'strange', 'mad', 'insane', 'psycho', 'being silly' or 'needing a looney bin'. Meg thought she was going 'insane' when she developed the symptoms of PND. She described the barrier that was created between her and the outside world when she developed depressive symptoms:

> One night Caiden [partner] got home from work and I said, "Oh, I think I've got postnatal or something, there's something not right"... I didn't feel myself. I felt weird, disorientated, like I wasn't me at all. I'd get anxiety and panic attacks every ten minutes and then I thought I was going insane. And then I'd con myself I was insane and then I was scared to go out the house.

Nicky rejected the 'unfair label' of PND as she had 'so many other contributing factors'. These factors included caring for her terminally ill mother during her second pregnancy, the death of her mother at her home after birth, struggling with a difficult toddler, and having financial difficulties. She discussed her experience:

> I had a real problem with the term postnatal depression because I felt that I had so many other contributing factors. I felt that it was an unfair label... but I realise now that depression is depression. Postnatal obviously because it occurs after the birth of a baby and that's when my depression did occur.

Kristina perceived there was stigma associated with the label of PND as it meant she was a 'terrible mother'. She suggested changing the name to 'postnatal disorder' to avoid the stigma of depression:

> It [PND] needs to be changed, it shouldn't be [called] postnatal depression. It should be postnatal disorder because the depression part sounds like you're not coping, you're a terrible mother. It was the stigma, that's why I didn't want anybody to know. I feel [sic] more comfortable with it the second time, but back then I was not comfortable admitting that [PND] to anybody, let alone go on antidepressants – no way!

The following quote by Thompson and colleagues (2004: 529) echoes the sentiments of many women in our study who experienced the lack of support from others and isolation as a result of the stigma of PND:

> The stigma of mental illness is increasingly recognised, with growing concern for the way it undermines social connectedness, social support, and opportunities for recovery.

The stigma of depression has been reported extensively in the literature (Brockington 1996; Brown et al. 1994; Buultjens and Liamputtong 2007; Mauthner 2002; Morrow et al. 2008). Similar to the findings from our study, Brown and associates (1994) revealed that one woman hid her depression from her maternal and child health nurse as she feared her baby would be taken away if she admitted she was depressed or not coping.

The stigma associated with the label of PND can contribute to feelings of being a failure. Brockington (1996) uses the term 'role failure' to describe the negative consequence of labelling with feelings of personal failure. The label of PND can also have a major impact on women's relationships with their partners, children, friends and extended family, particularly when others misunderstand the condition. Of importance is the need to identify women with PND who are clearly depressed so that treatment can be offered.

Feminist sociologists continue to challenge the label of PND, as they propose that the social context of motherhood makes women susceptible to depression. Since the 1960s, feminists have argued that the label of PND should be changed as it ignores the transitional process of early motherhood (Fullager and Gattuso 2002; Gammell and Stoppard 1999; Kitzinger 1992; Maushart 1997, 2005; Mauthner 2002; Nicolson 1990; Oakley 1992; Scattolon and Stoppard 1999). There is evidence in the literature that the label of PND needs to be changed to be more mother-friendly. In the United Kingdom, the term 'postnatal illness' is used to encompass a range of mood disorders after childbirth, including PND. Similarly, Oates (2003) asserts that unhappiness after childbirth is common and women may not necessarily be depressed. Along a similar vein, Matthey and colleagues (2002) suggest using the term 'postnatal mood disorder', instead of PND, to acknowledge the adjustment associated with having a baby.

The perceived stigma of mental illness deters many individuals from seeking help (Sirey et al. 2001) and contributes further to their low self-esteem, isolation and hopelessness (WHO 1999). The stigma of being diagnosed with a form of mental illness carries with it the connotation that the individual has 'a disturbance of mental functioning be it intellectual capacities, thought processes, emotions or underlying motivations' (Busfield 1996: 52). The stigma that individuals experience can have a deep and lasting impact (Hinshaw and Ciccetti 2000) at the time of diagnosis and even when individuals resolve the illness. This social stigma can also affect an individual's personal life, such as housing, employment and health insurance (Eriksen and Kress 2005).

6.2   Women's Experiences and Drawings of PND

The women were asked to discuss their experiences of PND to provide a contrast to the biomedical understanding of PND, and they were also asked to either draw or write a statement about it. In contrast to the predominant biomedical under-standing of PND, women commonly expressed findings, which are also revealed in the sociological literature, such as: feeling trapped (Beck 1992; Chan et al. 2002; Scattolon and Stoppard 1999; Sturman and Mongrain 2005), isolated from other mothers (McVeigh 1997; Paris and Dubus 2005; Scattolon and Stoppard 1999), feelings of despair (Beck 1992) and wanting to escape (Beck 1992; Gilbert and Allan 1998; Seligman and Rosenhan 1998). While we were unable to locate drawing as a means of depicting PND in the literature, Vincent Van Gogh has painted his experience of depression. Art is also used as a form of therapy in mental health (Perry et al. 2008).

Women's drawings were clear images of the darkness that represented their lived experience of PND. The darkness of their depression was not always evident from their interview descriptions. Postnatal depression represented a never-ending darkness where women perceived they were alone and where suicide was sometimes seen as providing a glimmer of hope to the misery they were experiencing. Women's drawings encompassed the feeling of being trapped alone in the dark. In this dark place, they experienced feelings of helplessness and despair. Compared with women's verbal accounts, their visual representations of PND captured more effectively their understanding of PND. Women's drawings provided a way of understanding women's inner feelings and emotions when they developed PND that were sometimes difficult to express during the interview.

6.2.1   Enveloping Darkness

Women's verbal accounts of PND and their drawings gave evidence of the enveloping darkness that the women experienced. However, the women's drawings of PND were far more powerful than their verbal accounts. Most of the women's drawings represented darkness, and they used the following metaphors when describing their drawings of PND: 'Everything just looks dark and covered with a black cloud', 'black hole', 'dark tunnel or hole', 'in a box', 'in a bubble', 'big, black bucket', 'totally black' and 'dark clouds all around me'. Similarly, women in Mauthner (2002) study reported PND as a dark hole, tunnel, prison, cage, box or pit. The women participants also discussed the feeling of being surrounded or enveloped in the darkness of their depression, which they described as 'always hovering', made them feel 'closed in' and 'never-ending'. One woman described how 'time couldn't go fast enough'. Women's sense of helplessness is evident from these drawings, as one woman stated that she was, 'groping [and] never really knowing what to do'. Similar findings of helplessness have been suggested by other researchers (see Brown et al. 1987; Gilbert and Allan 1998). Meg was one of the two participants who drew PND as total darkness (Fig. 6.1). She also added the words '[it's] never ending it's there day in and day out' at the top of the page. Meg described her drawing of PND:

> I did total black because it is horrible, it's never ending. It's a nightmare and couldn't add colour because there is nothing that's nice about it. You'd never want to have it again. It would be your worse nightmare, to me anyway.

Beatrice was also surrounded by darkness that she described as 'painful' and 'sharp'. Beatrice described her drawing of PND as darkness with lighter moments (Fig. 6.2):

> There's a sort of perspective that it's bearing down in on you and they're dark, painful, sharp shapes, dangerous pointy shapes that are like the thoughts that come in to you and hurt you. In between those sharp dangerous shapes and black moments there's what you might call

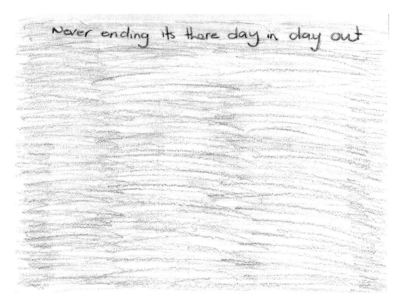

Fig. 6.1 Meg's image of PND

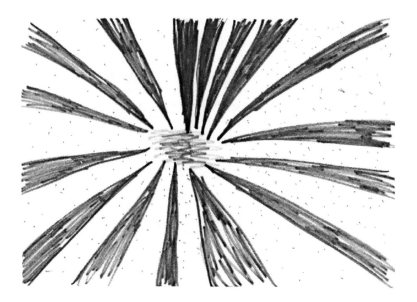

Fig. 6.2 Beatrice's image of PND.

lighter moments. They are like something you'd tip out of a vacuum cleaner bag, this grey senseless mass of particles that doesn't really make any sense. You can feel it on your mouth and on your skin. You want to shake it off you and it's there as a veil between you and everything else. You might objectively say that's a nice day, this is a lovely party, this is a special moment, [but] you still feel like you're separated by some sort of veil- dark, dusty, grey [and] senseless. It's as senseless as the particles in a vacuum cleaner.

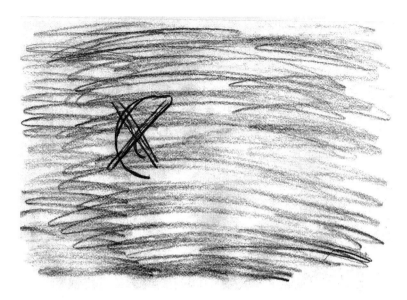

Fig. 6.3 Kristina's image of PND

Similar to Meg's image of PND, Kristina's drawing of PND was also of total darkness. Kristina felt trapped in the darkness that seemed inescapable. She drew an ear to represent the noise that she hated hearing when she was depressed (Fig. 6.3). When Kristina was asked to describe her drawing, she replied:

> I hated being myself. I hated who I was. It was just a dark, dark place I couldn't out of, and no matter how hard I tried I wanted to be out of this place [talking while drawing]. I just wanted to be happy again. I just wanted to be myself again. I wanted to be functional. I just could not get myself out of it. I just remember noise, I hated noise. It irritated me. Those are ears in case you didn't know [laughs]… It was just low noise, I just needed quiet. I couldn't stand it. I couldn't stand being around noise. I'm still a little bit like that now. I never used to be. If I'm under a bit of pressure, and I'm hearing it I get irritated by it.

6.2.2 Feeling Trapped and Alone

All of the women's drawings highlighted the feeling of being trapped and alone when they developed PND. Women's perceptions of inadequate support from others meant that women were struggling alone with little opportunity for rest or respite. The feeling that no one else could possibly understand their situation exacerbated women's feelings of isolation and aloneness. The women perceived they were confined to both motherhood and their PND, both of which seemed inescapable. Georgia drew a box to represent the sense of being trapped and the physical barrier between her and the outside world. In her drawing, Georgia is obviously sad and cocooned by her depression. When Georgia was asked to describe her drawing in Fig. 6.4, with tears in her eyes, she simply said, 'I'm in a box and I'm alone'.

Fig. 6.4 Georgia's
image of PND

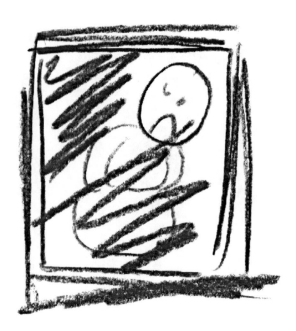

Fig. 6.5 Mary's
image of PND

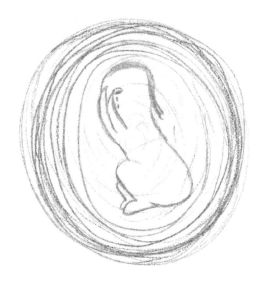

Similarly, Mary's drawing depicts the feeling of being trapped and isolated when she was depressed, as she perceived that no one understood what she was experiencing. Mary placed herself in a black hole rather than a box. Her description of her drawing (Fig. 6.5) was also brief:

> It's not a very good drawing. [I am] basically curled up, hands up to the eyes crying, in a black hole. **That's how you felt when you were depressed?** Yes…it's very hard to imagine anybody understanding what you're actually going through. You feel very alone, very misunderstood.

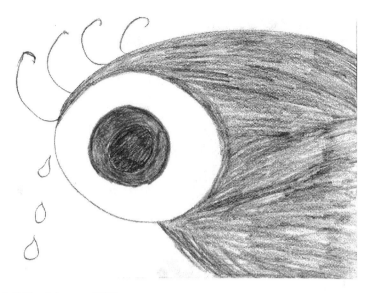

Fig. 6.6 Bridget's image of PND

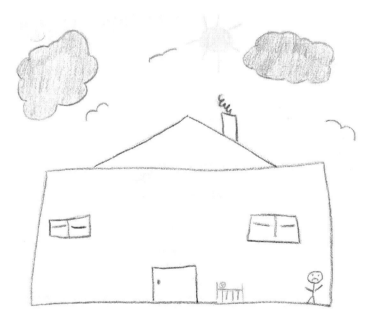

Fig. 6.7 Kelly's image of PND

Both Kelly (Fig. 6.7) and Georgia's (Fig. 6.4) drawings show a total disconnection from the outside world and a sense of confinement. These drawings provided a startling representation of women's lived experiences of PND.

Bridget's image of PND (Fig. 6.6) also highlighted the feeling of being alone and trapped. Bridget's drawing of PND was an eye filled with tears. She described her image as 'no light, it's an eye with tears, helpless, me looking at black'. Kelly, Georgia and Bridget's images are powerful portrayals of what PND was like for the female participants. It is clear to see how women would want to escape when they felt trapped and isolated from others.

Kelly's disconnection from the outside world was also evident from the description of her drawing (Fig. 6.7). In this drawing, Kelly is sad and trapped in a black house that represents her PND. Although Kelly's picture at first glance appears bright, her sadness and disconnection from the baby are evident in her drawing. She discussed how she felt emotionally trapped and detached from others, including the baby, when she experienced PND:

> [I am] inside, baby in cot away from me. [I am] sad. It's a nice day outside but I'm inside – feeling trapped, emotionally not physically. People walk past but I am not a part of life outside.

The link between depression and feeling trapped has been made in the literature (Brown et al. 1995; Craig 1996; Fournier et al. 2002; Gilbert and Allan 1998; Sturman and Mongrain 2005). Scattolon and Stoppard (1999) also revealed that depressed women felt trapped and alone. In their study, one woman perceived her depression to be like the isolation experienced in a jail cell. Gilbert (1989) used the term 'blocked escape' to describe depressed individuals who felt trapped and were unable to free themselves from an unrewarding environment. Not surprisingly, Brown and colleagues (1995) contend that women who felt trapped were three times more likely to develop depression.

Researchers have also found that women with PND feel trapped (Beck 1992; Chan et al. 2002; Mauthner 2002). Mauthner (2002) claimed that women with PND were imprisoned in their own misery of their depression. In the United States, Beck (1992) interviewed seven women with PND. In her phenomenological study, women felt trapped in their isolation, as they contemplated death as the only form of escape from their suffering. Chan and associates (2002) interviewed 35 Hong Kong Chinese women with PND who also felt trapped when they were unable to escape their situation. These women felt isolated from others and perceived that the lack of support from partners and in-laws contributed to their depressive symptoms. The women's desire for escape will now be discussed.

6.2.3 Escape

Most of the women wanted to escape from the darkness, isolation and confinement that represented motherhood and their PND. What was also evident from women's stories was the underlying perception of themselves as 'bad mothers'. Of the women who wanted to escape, almost half of them were suicidal – five had suicidal thoughts, one had suicidal plans, and two had attempted suicide. However, a small number of women who voiced not wanting to escape also had suicidal thoughts, but none of them had suicidal plans or attempts.

Kristina echoed the sentiments of many women in our study, as she desperately wanted to escape from her PND. Amidst the darkness of her PND were feelings of self-hatred, sadness and helplessness. Kristina explained her desperate need to escape from the darkness of her PND:

> I hated being myself. I hated who I was. It was just a dark, dark place I could not get out of, and no matter how hard I tried, I wanted to be out of this place. I just wanted to be happy again. I just wanted to be myself again.

Similarly, Meg wanted to escape from the darkness of her depression as it seemed too difficult to conquer. Her thoughts of escaping stemmed from her feelings of exhaustion and difficulty in overcoming PND. She remarked:

> Some days you wouldn't care if anything happened to you if you didn't wake up. You really wouldn't want it to happen but you'd think sometimes at night, oh if I didn't wake up it would be so much easier…It [PND] is a lot of hard work and energy to try and get over, some days when you haven't got it you think, I don't think I can do this. It would be so much easier if, I don't know, you could just disappear.

Bridget also wanted to escape even for a day from motherhood. For her, escape was a whimsical fantasy. Bridget was not suicidal, but imagined that everyone would be better off without her:

> You have thoughts where you just want to be away from this world for a day – like it's a fairyland sort of thing…you really don't want to be. You do have imaginings that this world could be better without me but you're not serious… I don't think I was suicidal but I definitely felt like I wanted to I don't know disappear I guess in a magical sort of way.

Kath, like Bridget, also perceived that her partner and children would be better off without her if she escaped from motherhood. She perceived herself as a 'hopeless' mother and wife. Intertwined with Kath's thoughts of hopelessness, she had fleeting thoughts of wanting to escape to the Bahamas:

> I just thought that everyone would be better without me. I wanted to get on a plane and go to the Bahamas… I was a hopeless mother, and a hopeless wife.

Similarly, Georgia wanted to go somewhere warm and tropical to escape the continual crying from her baby. The notion of escaping from motherhood provided a glimmer of hope and made her feel like she had some emotional control over the situation. She explained:

> I could just run away to Queensland… I think mentally I needed to feel like I had a choice. I needed to feel that there was some escape that I could make from hearing that baby cry all the time.

Diane also wanted to escape from motherhood as she perceived herself to be a 'bad mother' who was unable to cope with the demands of motherhood. Her quote describes the helplessness she felt when she was depressed. Diane wanted to escape motherhood as she felt obsolete. She discussed how her husband could artificially feed and care for their baby:

> I had this plan that I was going to take a bus to the airport…because I was such a bad mother. I would just leave them, and [my partner] would cope really well, so he could look after her, and put her on formula and she would be fine, and she doesn't need me.

Researchers have suggested that depressed individuals want to escape from their situation (Beck 1992; Carson and Arnold 1996; Gilbert and Allan 1998; Seligman and Rosenhan 1998). However, the meaning of escape has been poorly researched. In the literature, escape was first described in the learned helplessness model of depression. Edward (Bibring 1953) was the founder of the learned helplessness model. In more recent times, social rank theorists (Gilbert and Allan 1998) have developed this model. They theorise that failed attempts to escape result in a state of defeat. In our study, women also felt defeated when they wanted to escape from motherhood and their depressive symptoms.

There is evidence in the literature that women with PND want to escape from motherhood (Beck 1992; Chan et al. 2002; Jordan 1998; Kennedy et al. 2002; McIntosh 1993). Similar to the findings from our study, Beck (1992) claimed that women wanted to escape from their obsessive thoughts as they perceived they had failed at motherhood. McIntosh (1993) interviewed 60 first-time mothers in Scotland and also found that women wanted to escape from the confinement of motherhood. In the study by McIntosh (1993), one woman voiced, 'It's being stuck in the house... I just feel I want to go away and never come back sometimes'. In contrast to the findings from our study, Chan and colleagues (2002) found that women's only escape from motherhood was through violent means – homicide or suicide.

The notion of suicidal intent when individuals are depressed has been well documented in the literature (Beck and Indman 2005; Cox and Holden 2003; Kennedy et al. 2002; Stewart and Jambunathan 1996; Tam et al. 2002). Carson and Arnold (1996) in their book *Mental Health Nursing. The Nurse-Patient Journey* state that depressed individuals with thoughts of escape have a moderate risk for suicide. Carson and Arnold (1996) contend that 'the patient does not want to die, so much as escape from his sense of being overwhelmed by his problems... he feels like he is a 'burden to others'''. This definition of escape is not gender-specific. Carson and Arnold (1996) describe five levels of risk for suicide: no suicidal thoughts; mild thoughts of suicide (fleeting thoughts); moderate thoughts of suicide; advanced thoughts of suicide (suicide attempts) and severe thoughts of suicide (intrusive thoughts of death and the only solution is to suicide).

From these findings and the number of women in our study who fantasised about escaping, it is difficult to know if women who want to escape are more likely to contemplate suicide. The desire to escape and the risk of suicide need further investigation. It also needs to be explored using a clinical interview rather than a screening tool as it may provide valuable information about women's level of risk.

6.2.4 *Despair*

The notion of despair resulted from on-going feelings of helplessness and hopelessness where women could see no escape from their situation. The women who attempted suicide did so not to end their lives but to show others how desperate they were to get help. Their comments such as 'the thought that the kids wouldn't be able

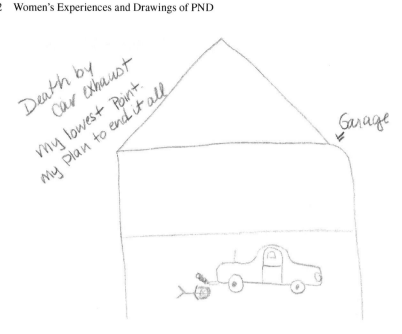

Fig. 6.8 Sue's image of PND

to cope without me' (Samantha) and 'these two little people needed me' (Georgia) concur with Cox and Holden (2003) findings that women with PND are unlikely to suicide because of the presence of others, particularly children. Alarmingly, however, most women commented how easily they could have 'crossed the line' and hurt themselves or their children when they experienced fleeting moments of irrational behaviour. Sue described her drawing (Fig. 6.8) as 'Death by car exhaust. My lowest point. My plan to end it all'. Her drawing epitomises the misery she was experiencing when she was depressed. Amidst these fleeting irrational thoughts were moments of rationality. During the interview, Sue discussed how she had ten different ways that were methodically planned to kill herself. She gave a chilling account of how she planned to end her life:

> Well the first [PND] picture was I guess what you could say [was] my lowest point of depression. I had about ten different ways to kill myself and the one that I kept going to, if I had followed through is this picture. My plan was to go downstairs into the garage of my now in-laws' house and run my mother-in-law's car with the garage door closed, and lay down next to the exhaust and go to sleep, never wake up. That was pretty much my plan. Death by car exhaust was pretty much what I named it because that was the whole plan. The scary thing is that I had actually gone down those stairs to follow through with that on more than one occasion and every time I'd just about get to the last stair and looking at the garage door thinking all I have to do is open it and start the car. Reality would come, what are you doing? This is not what's supposed to happen. So I would go back upstairs, eat more chocolate, and call my husband. He wasn't my husband then, call Tom and cry.

Barbara was also suicidal when she experienced feelings of despair. In a state of despair, she had feelings of helplessness and numbness when she developed PND.

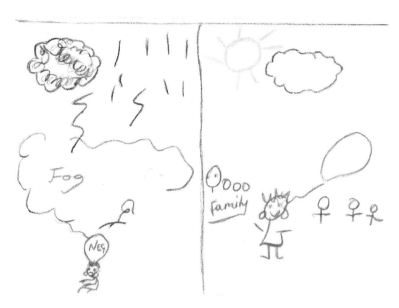

Fig. 6.9 Barbara's image of PND and resolution

She described her drawing (Fig. 6.9, which shows PND on the left and resolution on the right) of despair as 'being a vegetable' when she was depressed:

> It's all fog, and dark and negative. It was like trying to work your way through a pitch black fog, and groping- never knowing really what to do. Just a horrible [feeling], not wanting to be alive really. **Feeling like you couldn't get out of it?** Yes, just despair- absolute despair, but worse than despair if you could be worse than despair… To me it's like being a vegetable, because your mind's not working but you're there in person. You're just working on a go button that says, "Feed this. Do that. Do this"- that's all it was.

It is well documented in the literature that depressed individuals experience feelings of defeat, hopelessness and humiliation (Bibring 1953; Brown 1998; Gilbert and Allan 1998). However, there have been no visual accounts of the despair that women with PND experience. In the United States, Beck (1992) found an association between women's deep levels of depression and suicidal thoughts. Beck (1992) argued that suicidal thoughts provided a sense of escape for women and an end to the nightmare of motherhood. From a different perspective, Nahas and Amasheh (1999) claimed that no suicidal ideation was reported in a qualitative study of Jordanian mothers living in Australia; perhaps this was because these women were not severely depressed. The difference in findings could also be due to cultural and religious practises.

6.3   Chapter Summary

This chapter has explored women's experiences of PND. Some women admitted to lying or being dishonest when they completed the EPDS to preserve their image of being 'good mothers'. The majority of women perceived that their PND occurred as a result of their circumstances and the lack of support from others. Secondly, their perception of PND as a severe disorder meant that milder forms of the illness did not exist. Of interest, partners were more likely to agree with the diagnosis of PND. Of importance, the term 'postnatal' was used by the participants when they talked about PND. Perhaps this meant that couples had difficulty in labelling PND as depression.

What was evident from the couples' stories was the range of psychosocial factors they saw as contributing to depressive symptoms. Women perceived they were trapped in the motherhood role and in the darkness of their depression. The feeling of entrapment resulted in thoughts of wanting to escape, which provided a glimmer of hope from the constant demands of motherhood and the all-encompassing darkness that represented PND. The following feelings were common from women's stories around the time of diagnosis: feeling so different that they were socially isolated; feeling so inadequate that they could no longer keep up the façade; feeling so ashamed as they were unable to cope with being a mother; feeling so trapped in their helplessness that they were unable to escape and feeling so tired that mustering up the energy made escape seem impossible. Women's drawings of PND highlighted the feeling of being trapped alone in the dark when women were depressed and resulted in feelings of despair and helplessness.

In the next chapter, we will explore the partners' experiences of PND and the impact of PND on the partner and the couple's relationship.

References

Beck, C. T. (1992). The lived experience of postpartum depression: A phenomenological study. *Nursing Research, 41*(3), 166–170.

Beck, C. T., & Indman, P. (2005). The many faces of postpartum depression. *Journal of Obstetric, Gynecologic, and Neonatal Nursing, 34*(5), 569–576.

Beyond Blue. (2006). What is postnatal depression? http://www.beyondblue.org.au/index.aspx?link_id=94. Accessed 12 June 2007.

Bibring, E. (1953). Mechanisms of depression. In P. Greenacre (Ed.), *Affective disorders: Psychoanalytic contributions to their study.* New York: International Universities Press.

Brockington, I. (1996). *Motherhood and mental health.* Oxford: Oxford University Press.

Brown, G. W. (1998). Genetic and population perspectives on life events and depression. *Social Psychiatry and Psychiatric Epidemiology, 33,* 363–372.

Brown, G. W., & Harris, T. (1978). *Social origins of depression. A study of psychiatric disorder in women.* London: Tavistock Publications Limited.

Brown, G. W., Bifulco, A., & Harris, T. O. (1987). Life events, vulnerability and onset of depression: Some refinements. *The British Journal of Psychiatry, 150,* 30–42.

Brown, S., Lumley, J., Small, R., & Astbury, J. (1994). *Missing Voices. The experience of motherhood.* Melbourne: Oxford University Press.

Brown, G. W., Harris, T. O., & Hepworth, C. (1995). Loss, humiliation and entrapment among women developing depression: A patient and non-patient comparison. *Psychological Medicine, 25*(1), 7–22.

Busfield, J. (1996). *Men, women and madness. Understanding gender and mental disorder.* London: MacMillan.

Buultjens, M., & Liamputtong, P. (2007). When giving life starts to take the life out of you: Women's experiences of depression after childbirth. *Midwifery, 23,* 77–91.

Carson, V. B., & Arnold, E. N. (1996). *Mental health nursing. The nurse-patient journey.* Philadelphia: W.B. Saunders.

Chan, S. W. C., Levy, V., Chung, T. K. H., & Lee, D. (2002). A qualitative study of the experiences of a group of Hong Kong Chinese women diagnosed with postnatal depression. *Journal of Advanced Nursing, 39*(6), 571–579.

Cox, J. L., & Holden, J. (2003). *Perinatal mental health. A guide to the Edinburgh Postnatal Depression Scale (EPDS)*. London: Gaskell.

Craig, T. K. J. (1996). Adversity and depression. *International Review of Psychiatry, 8,* 341–353.

Eriksen, K., & Kress, V. E. (2005). *Beyond the DSM story*. Thousand Oaks: Sage.

Fournier, M. A., Moskowitz, D. S., & Zuroff, D. C. (2002). Social rank strategies in hierarchical relationships. *Journal of Personality and Social Psychology, 83*(2), 425–433.

Fullager, S., & Gattuso, S. (2002). Rethinking gender, risk and depression in Australian mental health policy. *Australian e-Journal for the Advancement of Mental Health, 1*(3), 1–13.

Gammell, D. J., & Stoppard, J. M. (1999). Women's experiences of treatment of depression: Medicalization or empowerment? *Canadian Psychology, 40*(2), 112–128.

Gilbert, P. (1989). *Human nature and suffering*. London: Lawrence Erlbaum.

Gilbert, P., & Allan, S. (1998). The role of defeat and entrapment (arrested flight) in depression: An exploration of an evolutionary view. *Psychological Medicine, 28*(3), 585–598.

Hinshaw, S. P., & Ciccetti, D. (2000). Stigma and mental disorder: Conceptions of illness, public attitudes, personal disclosure, and social policy. *Development and Psychopathology, 12,* 555–598.

Holopainen, D. (2002). The experience of seeking help for postnatal depression. *Journal of Advanced Nursing, 19*(3), 39–44.

Jordan, M. (1998). Report in International Herald Tribune, September 7th, p. 8.

Kennedy, H. P., Beck, C., & Driscoll, J. W. (2002). A light in the fog: Caring for women with postpartum depression. *Journal of Midwifery and Women's Health, 47*(5), 318–330.

Kitzinger, S. (1992). *Ourselves as mothers. The universal experience of motherhood*. London: Doubleday.

Matthey, S., Kavanagh, D, Howie, P., Barnett, B., Charles, M. (2002). Prevention of postnatal distress or depression: an evaluation of an intervention at preparation for parenthood classes. Journal of Affective Disorders 79(1–3): 113–126.

Maushart, S. (1997). *The mask of motherhood*. Sydney: Random House.

Maushart, S. (2005). *What women want next*. Melbourne: Text Publishing.

Mauthner, N. S. (2002). *The darkest days of my life. Stories of postpartum depression*. Cambridge: Harvard University Press.

McIntosh, J. (1993). Postpartum depression: Women's help-seeking behaviour and perceptions of cause. *Journal of Advanced Nursing, 18,* 178–184.

McVeigh, C. (1997). Motherhood experiences from the perspective of first-time mothers. *Clinical Nursing Research, 6*(4), 335–348.

Milgrom, J., Martin, P. R., & Negri, L. M. (1999). *Treating postnatal depression. A psychological approach for health care practitioners*. Chichester: Wiley.

Morrow, M., Smith, J., Lai, Y., & Jaswal, S. (2008). Shifting landscapes: Immigrant women and post partum depression. *Health Care for Women International, 29*(6), 593–617.

Nahas, V. L., & Amasheh, N. (1999). Culture care meanings and experiences of postpartum depression among Jordanian Australian women: A transcultural study. *Journal of Transcultural Nursing, 10,* 37–45.

Nicolson, P. (1990). Understanding postnatal depression: A mother-centred approach. *Journal of Advanced Nursing, 15,* 689–695.

Oakley, A. (1992). *Social support and motherhood. The natural history of a research project*. Oxford: Blackwell.

Oates, M. R. (2003). Postnatal depression and screening: Too broad a sweep? *The British Journal of General Practice, 53,* 596–597. August.

Paris, R., & Dubus, N. (2005). Staying connected while nurturing and infant: A challenge of new motherhood. *Family Relations, 54,* 72–83.

Perry, C., Thurston, M., & Osborn, T. (2008). Time for me: The arts as therapy in postnatal depression. *Complementary Therapies in Clinical Practice, 14,* 38–45.

Scattolon, W., & Stoppard, J. M. (1999). "Getting on with life": Women's experiences and ways of coping with depression. *Canadian Psychology, 40*(2), 205–219.

Seligman, M. E., & Rosenhan, D. L. (1998). *Abnormality.* New York: W.W. Norton & Company.

Shakespeare, J., Blake, F., & Garcia, F. (2003). A qualitative study of the acceptability of routine screening of postnatal women using the Edinburgh Postnatal Depression Scale. *The British Journal of General Practice, 53,* 614–619. August.

Sirey, J. A., Bruce, M., Alexopoulos, G. S., Perlick, D. A., Friedman, S. J., & Meyers, B. S. (2001). Stigma as a barrier to recovery: Perceived stigma and patient-rated severity of illness as predictors of antidepressant drug adherence. *Psychiatric Services, 52,* 1615–1620.

Stewart, S., & Jambunathan, J. (1996). Hmong women and postpartum depression. *Health Care for Women International, 17,* 319–330.

Sturman, E. D., & Mongrain, M. (2005). Self-criticism and major depression: An evolutionary perspective. *The British Journal of Clinical Psychology, 44*(4), 505–519.

Tam, L. W., Newton, R. P., Dern, M., & Parry, B. L. (2002). Screening women for postpartum depression at well baby visits: Resistance encountered and recommendations. *Archives of Women's Mental Health, 5,* 79–82.

Thompson, V. L. S., Noel, J. G., & Campbell, J. (2004). Stigmatization, discrimination, and mental health: The impact of multiple identity status. *The American Journal of Orthopsychiatry, 74*(4), 529–544.

Ugarriza, D. N. (2002). Postpartum depressed women's explanation of depression. *Journal of Nursing Scholarship, 34*(3), 227–233.

Whitton, A., Warner, R., & Appleby, L. (1996). The pathway to care in post-natal depression: Women's attitudes to post-natal depression and its treatment. *The British Journal of General Practice, 46,* 427–428.

WHO. (1999). Postpartum care of the mother and newborn: A practical guide. *Birth, 26*(4), 255–258.

Chapter 7
Living with Uncertainty: The Partners'
Experiences of Postnatal Depression

It got to the point where I'd actually pull up out the front [of the house] and listen- turn the radio off, turn the car off and listen before I actually got out the car just to see how things were at home because Alex wasn't an easy baby- he wasn't sleeping… I could tell if Alex was up crying and screaming that it wasn't going to be a very pleasant night (William).

[The] frantic phone calls- they were hard to handle… it was real desperation stuff like, "the kids are in the car. I'm going to kill them"… It was more verbal steam letting off, so I'd just let it go… I didn't think she would. I made it very, very clear that if I ever noticed anything that would be it- she knew without a doubt, because you've got to put the kids before anybody else… Nothing like that happened so that was good (Brian).

'Living with uncertainty' encompassed the men's experiences of living with PND. Most partners, like William and Brian, were living with uncertainty as they tried to cope with the stress at home due to women's unpredictable moods related to PND. This chapter will highlight the need to support the partners when women are diagnosed with PND. The partners were the main avenue of support for women when they developed PND. However, many partners in our study had difficulty providing support as they were experiencing distress or depression themselves, were working long hours or were unaware of the support women needed.

Our aim in this chapter is to explore the impact of PND on the partner. This chapter will identify the type of support that men need in the postpartum period for their emotional well-being. The chapter will highlight the challenges that men experienced as fathers and when their partner was diagnosed with PND. It will also examine the couple's relationship when women are depressed.

7.1 Living with Uncertainty: The Partners' Experiences of PND

Living with uncertainty captured the men's experiences of living with someone with PND, and their fears about whether or not they would find their wife or children dead. Women became resentful, irritable and angry as they struggled to cope with

C. Westall and P. Liamputtong, *Motherhood and Postnatal Depression: Narratives of Women and Their Partners*, DOI 10.1007/978-94-007-1694-0_7, © Springer Science+Business Media B.V. 2011

the burden of caring for the children. When men were unable to 'fix the problem' [PND], they spent longer at work to protect their sanity. Many of the partners struggled with depression themselves or struggled to cope with the uncertainty of day-to-day life. Ethan, like most of the partners, was living with uncertainty when his wife, Tara, was depressed:

> I had the batten down the hatches approach- just try and roll with the punches which is an expression you use, but roll with it and try and do anything to help- go out or do anything. And that was very difficult you know because you were never quite sure how she was going to react. She could be annoyed over something, and sometimes she reacted quite strongly... A couple of times I came home and she [Tara] was sitting on the couch almost catatonic with Rose [daughter] crawling around on her, or [she] just sits on the floor.

Ursula expressed her husband's shock when he found that she was no longer able to cope with the baby:

> My husband just went "Oh my God" and freaked out when he came home. I was sitting on the floor just in tears. Vicky [daughter] was going, "Mummy, it's okay mummy". I just couldn't handle it anymore.

Nicky told us about her husband's fear of finding her dead:

> Every now and then it would get a little bit hard for him to bear. And it got to the point where it was hard for him to always come home, and as he said in his own words one day, "I don't know whether I'm coming home to my wife alive or dead"... When he was really worried about me he would call me quite a lot. He'd ring his mum. He would reach out. Sometimes it brought him down when he always would come home to me upset.

In our study, all of the partners were male. Only one woman was single when she was diagnosed with PND. Two women were in relationships where there was domestic violence, and one of these relationships resulted in divorce. Two couples temporarily separated when women were depressed, and another couple divorced. Two other couples were dealing with legal battles and ongoing stress from blended relationships. As previously stated, in our study, women were the primary caregivers for their children. Similar to the women's experiences, the adjustment to fatherhood influenced men's sense of identity as well as their emotional well-being. Fletcher et al. (2006: 481) aptly capture the adjustment to fatherhood for first-time fathers in the following quote:

> The birth of his first child marks one of the most profound changes a man can undergo, transforming his standing in the community, his intimate relationships and his identity... It is important for the father to be ready to provide care and sustenance and to support the mother in her new role, but it is also important for him to have the mental and emotional resources needed to form a secure and nourishing relationship with his child.

We also found that the above quote was relevant not only for first-time fathers but also for fathers with two or three children.

Men have largely been ignored from studies investigating PND (Condon et al. 2004). As previously discussed, only three qualitative studies were located that examined the experiences of male partners of women who were diagnosed with

PND (Davey et al. 2006; Kowalski and Roberts 2000; Meighan et al. 1999). In an American study, Meighan and colleagues (1999) individually interviewed eight male partners and identified the following themes: she becomes an alien; he attempts to fix the problem, he makes sacrifices, loss of control, loss of intimacy, altered relationship and postpartum depression is a real thing – a crisis. In their study, the men also experienced fear and confusion and were concerned about their partner and felt they were unable to help them overcome PND. Most of the men in Meighan et al.'s study (1999) made sacrifices to keep the family together and were uncertain about their future with their wife who seemed like another person. Meighan and associates (1999) concluded that health professionals need to provide information to couples in antenatal classes and prior to discharge from hospital. Also to give the partners strategies if PND develops, as men influence women's recovery from PND. Davey and others (2006) conducted a focus group with 13 male partners of women who had been diagnosed with PND in Australia. They found that male partners were overwhelmed, isolated, stigmatised and frustrated when women developed PND. In the United Kingdom, Kowalski and Roberts (2000) undertook three unstructured 2-hours sessions with five male partners. They showed that the sessions benefited men as they were able to express their emotions, gained a better understanding of women's emotional needs and were given strategies to support women.

7.1.1   Difficulty Providing Support

Researchers have identified that the partners are an important source of support for women in the postnatal period (Beck 1996; Boyce 2003; Brown et al. 1994; Champion and Goodall 1994; Chan and Levy 2004; Dennis and Ross 2005; Kitzinger 1992; Mauthner 2002; Milgrom et al. 1999; O'Hara and Swain 1996). However, these studies failed to include the partners' perspectives. Our findings contrast those of Morse, Buist and Durkin (2001) who claimed that most women perceived their partners to be caring and loving in the postnatal period. However, the women in their study were not all diagnosed with PND.

In our study, the partners were the main source of support for women after the birth. However, most women were disappointed with the amount of emotional and practical support they received from their partner. The partners had difficulty providing support as they were either experiencing distress or depression themselves or had a poor understanding of PND. Morrow and associates (2008) suggested that a lack of awareness of PND among husbands of women with PND contributed to the lack of emotional support. Berggren-Clive (1998) claimed that women's expectations of support were often unfulfilled, particularly with the amount of support that partners provided. Furthermore, partners and family failed to provide the support that women needed, and consequently, women were lonely and deprived of a support network. George (1996) found, from his clinical experience, that partners influenced women's recovery from PND as they failed to understand the condition and were unaware of the support women needed. Katie, like many of the women in our study, expressed how her partner had difficulty understanding PND:

> I really don't think my partner understood that I had postnatal depression. Looking back I don't think he was all that compassionate about it through probably misunderstanding. There was a real lack of communication there of the condition.

Monica also expressed similar sentiments:

> As much as my husband was supportive, he didn't understand. And I still to this day don't think he understood what I went through. He's the kind of person who thinks, "Oh yes it was tough, let's move on"… Even when I was ringing him, and saying, "I'm walking around the house in circles, getting closer and closer to walls nursing this baby, thinking I could just bump his head could you come home please, he still didn't see the sense of urgency in what I was saying.

Marcia and Monica commented on the mismatch between the support women needed and the support they received from their partners:

> Everything he tried to do to help me was wrong, and I was getting really, really angry about everything. He found it hard to be sympathetic (Monica).

> We had people coming over a couple of weeks ago, and I said to him, "Can you just help me so I don't get stressed out?" And he went out and mowed the paddock! And I just thought, you've just got no idea, I needed practical help (Marcia).

Women were also the main source of support for their partners. Although the participants were interviewed separately, the partners' stories matched the women's accounts regarding the lack of support provided by the male partners. This finding suggests that women's perceptions of partner support were accurate. Unsupportive partners were described by women as persons lacking understanding, ignoring them when they were depressed, spending long hours at work or were away for days or weeks at a time. Women used the following words to describe their partners: 'never takes time off', 'unable to come home' and 'away a lot'. The long working days meant that the partners were unavailable to offer the support that women needed, namely, practical and emotional support. It was clear from the partners' stories that there was a tension between family and work commitments, as Kevin and Brian stated:

> I go out and make sure we have money but unfortunately it means Sarah doesn't then get the support that I'd want (Kevin).

> Being the breadwinner, if I fail we're in trouble… we fail financially as a family, and that does bring a lot of pressure on families (Brian).

The feeling of guilt was evident from many of the partners' stories as they blamed themselves for women's PND. Noah, a father of three, worked 12–14 h a day and was not available to offer the emotional and practical support that his partner needed. He started to blame himself for his partner's PND as he worked long hours:

> I'm a truck driver and I was working twelve to fourteen hours a day. I wonder to myself, am I the cause [of PND] because I'm away from the house so much? So she's not getting the normal support that probably other women get, so I started to think is it because of my job?

One partner from the focus group, Nick, also expressed feelings of guilt when he was away from home for most of the year:

> I thought it maybe was a reflection of my behaviour why she ended up like this [depressed] because I was traveling six to seven months out of the year, interstate, right and I started to blame myself for it.

The partners commonly expressed the demanding roles that women face as mothers. Tim spoke about the intensity of women's roles and the difficulty juggling child care with house work:

> You can see how women could be more vulnerable to depression if the guy is out all day… Being at home it's hard to cope… Just trying to juggle the kids and keep the house tidy, let alone cook meals and do washing.

The male partners fell into two groups – those that instinctively knew how to provide practical support and those that needed to be told what to do. Similarly, in their study, Andreason and Andreason (1990) contended that partners of women with twins fell into two groups – those who instinctively knew what to do to assist women with parenting and those who assisted women with parenting when problems arose, which meant that women were mainly responsible for child care and household chores. However, in our study, most women had difficulty verbalising their needs, and as a result, the practical and emotional support they needed was not provided. Beatrice expressed the difficulty she had accessing support from her partner when she was unable to express her needs:

> Although one thing that [partner] doesn't have is an ability to just listen, that perhaps a woman would have. Women will sometimes just sit and listen, while a lot of men tend to think, well, tell me what to do. Sometimes you can't tell them what to do- you don't know, but sometimes maybe you just want to talk about it. He does fall into the "tell me what to do" category and I'll do it, and that wasn't realistic or possible.

The partners openly discussed the lack of support they provided:

> A lot of my support was not supporting her- I didn't do anything. She was not receptive, so I basically didn't do anything. I had to do that to keep sane myself… There are no rules or regulations here- just fought your way through the dark as well… The greatest power you have is just walking away from something like that. It took me a long time to realise (Brian).

> I'd just sit back watching telly [television]. I didn't want to make small conversation. I'd just sit and watch the telly because she [partner] would go off [get upset]. I couldn't be bothered making the effort (Neil).

> On the weekends I'd just slump in the couch and stare at the telly. I would try and do lots around the house and projects (Liam).

The type of support women needed is highlighted in the following quotes by couples:

> I couldn't have got through it without him. I'd call him a couple of times a day or he'd call me just to see how I was going. I'd be calling over the stupidest things, little things. He was really good. David [partner] has always been fantastic, he has always been in there bathing, feeding [and] changing [baby] (Kim).

I do try and do my bit around the house with housework... and I guess I probably didn't make enough effort, but you've got to make an effort and really do those sorts of things because... if the house was untidy that was another thing playing on... Bridget's mind you know. "I've got to clean...but I've also got to bath the baby, and do this, this, this and this, and all these things are driving me mad". I'm not perfect but I did try to do more of that stuff to get it out of her hair (Ned).

Many of the partners, like Kyle, assisted women to treatment, as Maria said:

It wasn't until Kyle said, "I think you've got postnatal depression" which seemed silly, but after that [I thought], "you're right, you're right".

7.1.2 Work as an Escape

Most men openly admitted to spending more time at work to escape the turmoil at home as they had difficulty understanding and supporting women when they were depressed. As a result, women received limited support and were struggling with the bulk of child care and domestic duties. One partner in a study by Davey and colleagues (2006) worked longer hours, but this has not been reported as a common theme in the literature. Work became a safe haven for the partners and is reflected in the following quotes by Neil, William and Luke:

There were times I was just happy to get to work for a bit of peace and serenity, I was happy to get away (Neil).

You even got to the point even prior to getting home- you would find things to do at work to give you that five or ten minutes before you get home. There's nothing pleasant about walking into a tornado every night, and as much as you want to be there... sub-consciously you seem to lag back at work, even though you're not doing anything constructive- you may be just caught in a conversation... and it just becomes a habit (William).

There were times there you thought, "I'll stay here [at work] and start typing on my computer", which is terrible... but it was quite difficult for a while (Luke).

For some partners, although spending longer hours at work, they also voiced that this was less productive. Brian discussed how his day was longer as he had difficulty functioning at work as a result of sleep deprivation:

[Sleep deprivation is] very difficult to manage. You're not working at one hundred percent capacity so things take longer, so it all snowballs...It lengthens your day so then you come home later, and it's less help for Nancy [partner]... so that's how I've been coping by just doing longer hours to produce the same amount of work.

As men worked long hours, women voiced the need to contact men during the day to listen to their concerns. However, men found that the phone calls affected their performance at work. Liam, a doctor and a father of one, had difficulty concentrating on his job as he was receiving frequent phone calls from his partner:

She wasn't coping- you could see that. I was going to work, and I was waiting for phone calls- I couldn't concentrate on my job. It was terrible.

Similarly, one man from the focus group, Nick, discussed the call from his suicidal wife when he was interstate for business:

There was one time I flew to Perth to present the second largest contract I was working on. She rings up that night and says, "I feel like I'm going to suicide". You think do you just fly back now? I said, "Are you sure? Otherwise I'll hop on the plane now". She said, "No, no, I think I might be okay"… I said, "Look I can come back now. I can come back now". She said, "I think I'll be okay".

Several partners accessed support from work colleagues, and this was particularly beneficial to partners with limited support. Luke explained:

I didn't get any outside support or anything like that. You'd talk to friends at work [with kids]… so you'd bounce some ideas off each other…That was probably one of the better outlets.

Nathan in the focus group too said:

I told my boss, "my wife's got postnatal depression", and he said, "what do I need to do?" His wife had suffered depression… I said, "we can't afford to put the kids in day care" [so he paid for it once a week]… I just felt this massive relief when I told him.

7.1.3 The Emotional Well-being of Partners

In our study, several men openly discussed their past history of depression prior to women being diagnosed with PND, and a small number of men were diagnosed with depression when women received treatment for PND and were beginning to resolve symptoms. Of these partners, most sought help for their depression when they were suicidal. In their study, Meighan and colleagues (1999) also suggested that men suffered from the 'long lasting effects' of PND, even when women recovered. In our study, it is possible that the partners, who developed depression after the birth, were depressed at the same time as the women as they were also adjusting to parenthood and often had the same triggers such as sleep deprivation and the lack of support. Kyle, a mental health nurse with chronic depression, described the paradox of wanting to support his partner but at the same time needing support himself:

I had a great deal of difficulty supporting her because I was only just holding myself up. I just didn't want to have to support her as well.

Kyle's partner, Maria, described the impact of PND on her husband's emotional well-being and the see-sawing of emotions:

It took me a few months to feel like I can almost take on the world again, and then he dropped his bundle.

Lex discussed how he had difficulty coping when his wife was depressed, and how he could have been more supportive at the time:

I don't think I coped well overall, I got very, very angry with Diane, and I don't think I coped with it very well in retrospect. I guess I could have been a bit more supportive and understanding that this is something beyond her control, and that she can't snap out of it … I think I could have dealt with it better.

Lex, Diane's partner, remarked that:

Once he got really angry with me when I was crying. Then after that he was really helpful. I think it was hard for him to deal with, but since then he's been great he went with me to the doctor. I knew I could always talk to him about how I felt.

In their study, Meighan and colleagues (1999) also claimed that the men often realised they were depressed when they lived through women's depression. In our study, Melissa's husband stayed strong for her when she was depressed, but he was later diagnosed with depression and treated with antidepressants when she was on the road to recovery:

I just thought that I would mention that once I was off my antidepressants Paul [my partner] went on [antidepressants]. He was really strong for me... I guess in a way he was really strong for me for quite a while, and then when I was really turning the corner and coming off things he got really low... the loss of interest, the lack of motivation that sort of thing. He's gone on antidepressants, but he hasn't talked to a psychiatrist or a psychologist.

The importance of fathers as role models for the men was evident from many of the men's interviews. Kevin held himself together through his wife's PND because he wanted to be 'strong' like his dad. He was diagnosed with depression when his wife resolved PND. At this point, Kevin was suicidal and drinking heavily. He felt a gradual build up of depression over a 6 month period. During this time, he was separated from his wife for 1 month as he was unable to cope with being at home and was drinking heavily and getting into fights at the pub. Kevin reflected back on his experience of depression:

I held it together through that stuff [Sarah's PND] because that's what my dad did- he was strong, strong... You can be as macho as you like but you can snap just the same... It [depression] probably built up over six months... I actually went to the doctors... As doctors do [he] said, "Oh, you can have some valium"- which I took one, I've still got a packet of forty-nine. I went nuts for a while and I disappeared. I was drifting away from Sarah [partner] and just not wanting to go home... I didn't want to go home because it was getting ugly... I got into some fights, and I probably drank too much.

Sarah, Kevin's partner, also told us that:

We've had problems since which we traced back to that time. Kevin had, about a year and a half [to] two years ago he almost had a breakdown. He said it definitely started when I was going through my stuff [PND].

Kyle hid his depressive symptoms from his boss and his depressed wife for 15 months. He finally sought help for his depressive symptoms when he was suicidal:

I was still covering up my own depression, pretending I wasn't depressed... My boss said I'm not performing very well, and I think that was one of the triggers for me trying to kill myself, because I knew I wasn't performing well. I'd been trying to cover it [depression] up for about fifteen months... Within two weeks I had a counsellor and I was on Prozac.

Living with a depressed partner also affected men's emotional well-being. George (1996) contends that living with a depressed person contributes to depression as interactions are more negative, and cognition and problem solving abilities are decreased. One partner, Tim, discussed how living with a depressed partner affected his mood:

> Not having a real understanding of postnatal depression. I think it used to get me down you know, because I'd see her down- one minute she'd be up and then she'd be really flat and moody, I found that difficult too… I think it brought me down. I'm a fairly positive person, and when your partner's down it can bring you down too.

Some men used alcohol as a coping mechanism. Grant (1995) claims that men are more likely to abuse alcohol and drugs to cope with depression than women. Similar to the findings from our study, Cochran and Robanowitz (2003) suggested that paternal depression was associated with alcohol abuse and interpersonal conflict. Although in our study, interpersonal conflict was commonly experienced before the onset of depression in the partners. Ned, who was never diagnosed with depression, discussed using alcohol more frequently when he was 'run down, tired and frustrated'. He discussed how he put himself on the back burner when his wife was depressed:

> That's probably one thing I did more of- drink… I was getting run down, and tired and frustrated and everything else [pause]… that's basically how I coped with it- you just push everything aside and swear under your breath, and keep a happy face, and deal with everything, deal with yourself later. But I guess I never had to because you gradually come out of things, and that's all in the past now, so you just move on. But at the time you think just deal with it.

There is evidence in the literature that male partners also experience depression (Areias et al. 1996; Buist et al. 2002; Cochran and Rabinowitz 2003; Fettling 2002; George 1996; Goodman 2004; Matthey et al. 2000; Madsen and Juhl 2007; Paulson 2010; Ramchandani et al. 2005; Zelkowitz and Milet 1997, 2001). In their research, Buist and colleagues (2002) pointed out that male partners of depressed women have up to 50% higher rates of depression than partners of women who are not depressed. Goodman (2004) performed an integrative review to examine the rates of depression in partners of women with PND. The literature search from 1980 to 2002 was carried out using the CINAHL, PsychInfo and Medline electronic databases. Goodman (2004) located 20 studies and found that maternal depression was the strongest predictor of paternal depression in the postpartum period. During the first postpartum year, the incidence of paternal depression ranged from 1.2% to 25.5% in community samples and from 24% to 50% in men whose partners were experiencing PND.

Health services need to consider the emotional health of both partners when they are adjusting to parenthood (Buist et al. 2003; Currid 2005). Routine screening of women for PND needs to also include the partners. The EPDS has been validated to detect depression in English-speaking fathers in the postnatal period although different cut-off scores are recommended for men (ten or more) compared with women (13 or more) (Matthey et al. 2001). Matthey and others (2001) validated the EPDS in a sample of 208 fathers, using a cut-off score of over ten, they found 71.4% of depressed men and 93.8% of non-depressed men were correctly identified versus only 7% who were incorrectly identified. Goodman (2004) asserted that partners of women with PND need to be screened routinely in the postpartum period to lessen the risk to the child.

From our findings, the benefit of screening is to identify depressed partners, to offer early intervention and treatment and to improve the couple's relationship and to lessen the effects of depression on children.

7.1.4   Struggling to Understand PND

Most men had difficulty understanding PND as they were not included in treatment plans when women were diagnosed with PND. The partners wanted to receive information so they could understand PND and provide support to women to assist in their recovery. Being included in treatment plans would also provide an opportunity for the partners to be assessed for depression. In general, men had difficulty providing support as they felt helpless and had difficulty knowing how to support women. William succinctly discussed his lack of understanding about PND and how it contributed to the lack of support he was able to provide. He described the vague nature of PND and the potential for marital breakdown:

A lot of the conversation about how she was dealing with it and how she was feeling and all the rest of it...was about discussing it more with the female sex, not necessarily with the male sex, that may have been because she didn't have the confidence that I understood it. And that's another thing- if I don't understand it [PND] how am I supposed to support her? It's very difficult. I've never come across anything that's so vague. It's pretty hard to cope with so I don't know how the women cope with it... I can see how the marriage and partnerships can be broken down.

William's sentiments sum up the feelings of many other partners who felt helpless and frustrated when they struggled to understand PND and wanted to 'fix the problem':

Men can accept things when they can see the mechanics of something. There's something about hormones that they don't understand... We try and fix things, we don't go through a process we just fix them, and if we can't fix them we get confused and frustrated... As I said, it was very difficult to accept and understand because even when Kristina did try and explain to me [pause]- hormones. Isn't there a tablet to fix it? That's our answer? Isn't there something to correct your hormones, and to get you out of this depression?... How do you explain to someone that your hormones are out of whack, and that's what's causing you to behave this way? There's no logic. From a male perspective how do they try and assist someone through it when there's no real process to fix it? There's no real answer to it other than most probably finding out a little bit more about it medically. And maybe putting information sheets out in prenatal classes... and making males understand what the effect of hormones do to females, and I think that's maybe the catch cry. Even if we don't have a cure we can make people more aware of it, but we need to make people understand how the hormones actually work and what affect it has.

The difficulty in understanding PND created feelings of helplessness in the partners. Most partners felt helpless and ignored women when they were depressed as they were unable to 'fix the problem'. There is evidence in the literature that men want to 'fix the problem' when women develop PND (Brown et al. 1994; Fettling 2002; Mauthner 2002; Meighan et al. 1999). Meighan and colleagues (1999) similarly suggested that when men were unable to 'fix the problem', they became angry and frustrated. Brian discussed feeling helpless as he was unable to change his wife's irrational behaviour:

> It was hard… You look and you see the irrational behaviour and you just feel quite helpless. You just make suggestions or solutions and it's probably the worst thing you could do because they're not looking for solutions- they're looking for someone to vent at.

Most partners were not included in treatment plans when women were diagnosed with PND. They expressed the need to be included in treatment plans, rather than receiving written information, when women were initially diagnosed with PND. The dialogue in the men's focus group highlighted the exclusion of partners from treatment plans:

> Nick: This is the first group discussion we've had postnatally since it [PND] happened four years ago. I used to complain. Everything is about the woman, that's fine, but there's all these unresolved issues that have spun out of control as a result of that within the family. I wanted to get involved and be part of that, and also get some counseling too. It was not there.
>
> Michael: That's funny you say that because this is the first thing I've ever been to in relation to PND. I was, after our first [baby], a bit stressed, just the change in life that we went through [men agreeing] when you have your first baby. I think that probably didn't help, and I got a bit of [partner's] issues and things. As I've said this is the first thing I've ever been too.
>
> Nick: And the doctors took over, and the shrink took over. It was like, 'keep the husband out of the way, we want to take over!' [Everyone laughing]… Then I insisted with the shrink and I got involved.
>
> Michael: I don't think the GP's are qualified.
>
> Nathan: One really good thing about XXXX I felt quite involved I went to two sessions- they had two couple's nights which was really good. I felt a lot more involved in that process. I think that's really, really important. As you said, 'you're left in the dark'.
>
> Nick: No, they [health professionals] don't want you there either.

Several partners who were included in treatment plans were given information about PND and were also assessed emotionally by the health professional and some of them participated in group sessions specifically for the partners. The importance of including partners in treatment plans to increase their understanding of PND is highlighted in the following quotes:

> A lot of men don't know about postnatal depression or depression, and don't really understand it. I think going to the doctor's visits he [partner] saw how upset I was and he knew it [PND] must have been pretty bad (Meg).

> I felt like I needed it [father-baby unit!]… I went to see [the psychiatrist] a few times as well for me… because the stress was so high on me and so intense… It was very productive, and he and I decided, well he decided [laughs] I never thought I was depressed. We decided that I lead a highly stressed life and that sometimes I do dip into depression but I'm able to get myself out of it before it becomes a problem (Noah).

> I think the psychiatrist certainly did say, "well just bear with her and understand that it [PND] is not something you do just get over". And he did spend some time talking to me about what my perspective on it was and so on. And I think that was good for me to hear that as well, and to try to realise that she does need just time and support and that she's not herself- with time hopefully and the medication things should come good, and they did (Lex).

Partners who were not included in treatment plans voiced the need for more information about PND to be able to understand the condition, as Ned explained:

> I wasn't involved at all in any of the medical process, not for any of the follow up treatments or anything else. But certainly education is very important for anyone who's providing support to anyone with any kind of condition like that, and I think that was probably lacking... I think pamphlets are no good. "Come and see us by yourself- without your wife. Come and see us. Sit down and we'll have a chat. We'll go through some things". Give me some information- give me some tools and some skills to deal with it.

Ned continued about the need for partners to be given skills from health professionals to manage PND to assist women in their recovery:

> That's what I think is very, very important [that] anyone who has to support should be given some skills to do that, because they won't happen naturally. Just an understanding of what your partner's going through, and what you can do to help you know, or how or what you can do to cope with it. What you're likely to experience, and things like that to give you an understanding of what's going on, because you've got no idea. I think that would be really helpful to the support person which eventually helps the person themselves.

Several partners also gained a better understanding of PND when their partner experienced two or more episodes of PND. Kelly found that her partner was more supportive following her second episode of PND as he listened to her more:

> I found that I could talk to him and he'd listen, the second time around I think he listened more.

Diane told us that:

> I think he was the one that first picked it up, because I was crying all the time and he said, "Do you think you're depressed?" And I said, "No I don't think so, I'm just being silly" [laughs]. And even now I think he's still very sensitive- every time I say, "I'm a bit down today". "Do you think you're depressed? You need to go and see the GP".

Researchers have suggested that including men in support groups can improve the emotional well– being of both women and men. In an Australian study, Morgan and colleagues (1997) contended that a group program for postnatally distressed women and their partners decreased maternal distress and improved their self-esteem. The group intervention comprised of psychotherapeutic and cognitive-behavioural strategies over eight sessions. Half of the partners who attended the group sessions showed elevated levels of distress, but no explanation was given for this finding. Davey and associates (2006) conducted a 6-week group treatment with 13 male partners of women who had been diagnosed with PND, and a focus group was done at the end of the sessions to gain qualitative data. Davey et al. (2006) claimed that partners reported lowered levels of stress and depression after using a combination of psychoeducational and cognitive behavioural components and were more informed about PND. Matthey and the team (2004) conducted a randomised controlled trial that involved expectant partners in an antenatal class, and their results showed that when partners had an understanding of PND that women coped better with the emotional adjustment to motherhood.

7.1.5   The Stressed Relationship

Postnatal depression created a major wedge in the couple's relationship, and for most couples, resulted in the loss of intimacy. Researchers have found that relationship issues are common when women develop PND (Cox 2005; George 1996; Jeglic et al. 2005; Mauthner 2002; Meighan et al. 1999; Wilkinson and Mulcahy 2010). Meighan and colleagues (1999) revealed in their research that PND altered the couple's relationship and resulted in the loss of intimacy. The partners in our study reported increased levels of stress, frustration and anger as they were trying to cope with women's depressive symptoms. These emotions only added to the partners' feelings of helplessness. Increased stress was exacerbated by fatigue from ongoing sleep deprivation.

The partners used the following metaphors to describe their relationship: 'stressful', 'pressure', 'a lot of strain', 'tension', 'fighting' and 'conflict' when women were depressed. The partners discussed being 'on edge' and 'helpless' as PND was like a rollercoaster ride of emotions. Most of the male partners reported PND creating a 'wedge', 'a wall' or 'barrier' in the couples' relationships. William felt that PND caused a 'wedge' in his marital relationship. He discussed the lack of communication with his wife when she developed PND:

It's very difficult to work your way in when someone's got postnatal depression. You seem to get almost like a wedge between you and your family. It's not so much that it's being done intentionally- it's just the way you feel, and it's very difficult to cope with that as well as be [in] a supportive role.

Kevin made a poignant statement about the increased stress in his marital relationship contributing to his depression:

The effect of the stress at the time would cause me to have problems later on. Men are deeply affected by what their wives are going through.

Several women talked about the impact of PND on their marriage:

It [PND] probably put even more pressure on the marriage. We'd always had a bit of a rocky relationship and then when we had the children it probably only got worse. Probably because my attentions were more on the children and there's not as much time for the partner. That wasn't really tolerated that well. I think looking back if things were going along smoothly then my partner was okay- but once things got a bit rough and rocky the coping mechanisms weren't there (Katie).

I had a husband that kept telling me that he was going to leave me, and there was this part of my mind that said, "You should be trying to be more sexy, more bubbly, more attractive". But at the end of the day I had a baby that never stopped crying, and I had to stick my head down and look after my children... I didn't have the energy (Georgia).

Certainly our relationship at the time suffered significantly, so we were very distant. I remember Kyle...was also very depressed as well... I have always been the strong one. Once I was [depressed] too, who was there to hold us together and hold us up?... He was saying- not that we should split up- but that was what he was hinting at. The one thing I did know was that I wasn't going to lose him, so [pause] sex for us was certainly very painful after [the birth] for five to six months, so that was another thing that was niggling. I felt like my body was ruined (Maria).

Nevertheless, several participants, like Diane, felt that PND strengthened their relationship:

> I think it brought us closer, just because we've been through all this stuff together (Diane).

Partners used the expression 'walking on eggshells' when they described what it was like living with someone with PND. In their study, Morgan and colleagues (1997: 917) reported men's futile efforts to please their partners and the feeling they were 'treading on eggshells'. One partner in our study, Robert, discussed walking on eggshells and the increased stress on the relationship when his wife developed PND. When he was asked what their relationship was like at the time, he replied:

> [It was] very hard. You were walking on eggshells- you were tip toeing around situations... You finish work you come home, and Ellie dumps the baby and runs... if a confrontation came up I generally backed down and left it alone kind of scenario...when she was having a bad day... Generally, it would be an attack on anything I hadn't done for instance- it would be walk into the house and if I was three minutes late, "Why didn't you call?" If I was early it was, "The place is a mess. You don't help me around here". It would be anything, anything could trigger it off... and all of a sudden it was all your fault... maybe that was just an expression of anger that had to be pinpointed at someone or something.

Shane also discussed the relationship stress causing a feeling of uncertainty. As his wife was not receptive to communication, he described 'walking away' to protect his own sanity:

> [The relationship was] very stressful, not so much fighting but waiting to see what was going to happen next. It wasn't as if something terrible was going to happen, you just didn't know if there was going to be a fight or something like that. I felt on edge a little, just on edge... You didn't feel as if you were talking...In the heat of the moment you can say some terrible things and I'm guilty of that. It doesn't do any good at all... [I was] just on edge- trying to avoid an argument, and if one would start you'd pull your tongue in but it didn't always work.

Most men discussed the lack of sleep adding to the increased strain on the couple's relationship. Luke discussed the increased tension and sleep deprivation:

> Nothing you do seems to be right no matter how hard you try... I guess there was a lot of tension there- we fought about things whereas most of the time you wouldn't fight about it... I think particularly through that period it was tough, and probably goes back to the depression as well as the sleep deprivation- everything seems to be enhanced, and a disaster at the time... I could easily see how a couple could fall to pieces, and have separations... because it was the stress of the environment- it wasn't pleasant.

Tara remarked on the strain on her and her partner caused by her PND:

> It [PND] had this huge impact- suddenly I became this crazy woman, that's how I see it and he [Ethan] had to hold everything together. All of a sudden he had all this responsibility of the new baby and fending off well-meaning friends and relatives. And dealing with me just crying all the time, and saying I couldn't cope, and coming out with these ludicrous things. It's an enormous strain.

Most partners felt there was a lack of communication they experienced in their relationship as a result of PND because they had difficulty understanding women's distorted thought patterns. Lex had difficulty communicating with his wife because of her irrational behaviour and negative thoughts:

> I felt that it was very much one way communication, she wasn't talking and when she did she was quite irrational- she was on the verge [of being] psychotic- her depression was that bad… [Partner walked into the room]. Diane you were thinking completely irrational things- completely irrational [such as] "My family don't like her. My family doesn't want her there", all of these terrible things which were completely irrational. It's very hard to communicate with someone who's on the verge of being psychotic- she doesn't make sense of what she says. And you can tell her that it's not true, and she'll just revert into that same pattern of thought. So it's very much one-way communication.

The couple's relationship was also affected by the change in women's personalities as a result of PND. In their study, Meighan and colleagues (1999) used the category, 'she becomes an alien' to encompass the changes in women's personalities as a result of PND. After years of marriage and understanding his partner, William discussed how his wife was almost a stranger when she was depressed:

> You understand your partner, you understand their way of thinking, and that gets all thrown out the window [pause]… Obviously through courting [we] are linked- you end up understanding people- the way they react. And all that goes straight out the window, and you almost sometimes feel like you don't know the person. It's almost like a personality change.

Val talked about her feelings of being a stranger to her partner:

> I was not a very pleasant person to stay around and sometimes I wonder why he did because it was hard for him, I went from being so totally dependent on him to just so cross with him because I felt like he wasn't doing enough [stern voice], or supporting me enough, or whatever so he was in that situation where he couldn't lose- in the good books or in the bad books. You know there was no sex drive at all.

The loss of intimacy was commonly expressed by both partners when they reflected back on the impact of PND on their relationship. The need for intimacy in a relationship was evident from the men's stories and was reflected in the focus group interview:

> David: I wonder if it comes down to a good sexual relationship- part of being that bond together. I think once that got damaged then maybe there's more of a brick wall between. I reckon it's a big part of [a relationship].
> Nick: A big part of the depression is the libido. It's a statistical fact… Zoloft does it- suppresses.
> David: I found that me and [my partner] had a fairly good sexual relationship even through it [PND], you still found time to be together like that.

Nicky told us that due to the use of antidepressants, the sexual relationship between her and her partner had been affected greatly.

> I used to have quite a high libido and everything- that's all been numbed now [by Zoloft]. That's frustrating for me. I find he struggles a bit with it too because it's changed the way we used to be.

Nancy admitted similarly:

> I'm also on antidepressants [Zoloft] so that kills the libido and sometimes it's hard to reach orgasm. If we do happen to get together like that [intimately] he's just relieved that I want to [be intimate]. Yes, it is difficult because sometimes even though my body does yearn for it, I physically don't have the energy either and I really like to be left alone.

The treatment of PND focuses on the needs of women and not their partners (Fletcher et al. 2006). Matthey et al. (2004) provided a psychosocial intervention to expectant couples in routine antenatal classes to assess psychosocial adjustment of women and men after the birth. Preparation for parenthood classes were randomly allocated to one of three conditions: usual service ('control'), experimental ('empathy') or non-specific control ('baby play'). The intervention consisted of one separate antenatal class that targeted the psychosocial issues of first-time parents. The participants discussed possible postpartum concerns in separate gender groups, and then discussed these issues with their partners. Matthey et al. (2004) found that at 6 weeks postpartum women with low self-esteem, who received the intervention, were significantly better adjusted on measures of mood and sense of competence than women in the control groups. At 6 weeks postpartum, the partners of women were more aware of women's feelings, and women reported greater satisfaction with the sharing of household chores and childcare. Matthey and colleagues (2004) claimed that the brief and inexpensive intervention was effective in reducing postpartum distress in some of the first-time mothers. Davey and others (2006) conducted a 6-week group treatment program for male partners gave them the opportunity to share their experiences with others and provided strategies for improving their relationship and their emotional well-being. The program consisted of psychoeducational and cognitive behavioural components facilitated by two therapists.

There is evidence in the literature that women with PND perceive their partners to be unsupportive (Brown et al. 1994; Dennis and Ross 2005; Holopainen 2002; Kowalski and Roberts 2000; Mauthner 2002; Nahas et al. 1999; Wood et al. 1997). The lack of support from the partner can maintain women's PND (Boyce 1994; Dennis and Ross 2005; Matthey et al. 2003; Mauthner 2002; Milgrom et al. 1999; Misri et al. 2000). Dennis and Ross (2005) claimed that women who experienced a feeling of companionship and closeness to their partner were less likely to develop PND. Holopainen (2002) contended that women with PND felt unsupported by their partners when they failed to provide emotional and instrumental support. Mauthner (2002) found that women with PND received insufficient help from their partners even when women asked for help. In her study, women felt emotionally detached from their partners as they perceived their partners would be unable to understand their feelings. Brown and associates (1994) showed that most women with PND perceived their partners as unsupportive when they ignored their feelings and were unable to talk about PND. In an Australian study of ten women with PND who were admitted to a mother-baby unit, Buultjens and Liamputtong (2007) found that women attributed their depression to difficulties in their relationship with their partner. Although some of the partners provided practical support and assisted with childcare, women perceived them as unsympathetic to their feelings. Kowalski and Roberts (2000) conducted a 10-week closed group for women and three unstructured sessions with their partners. They found that women felt unsupported and contributed marital disharmony to their PND.

7.2 Chapter Summary

This chapter has examined the partners' experiences of PND and the support women and their partners need in the postpartum period. 'Living with uncertainty' captured the partners' experiences of living with someone with PND. When women developed PND, they needed support from their partners for their emotional well-being. However, many partners were experiencing distress or depression themselves or were not included in treatment plans to be given strategies to support women. In addition, most men were not included in treatment plans to learn about PND, were not assessed for depression or were not given strategies to support women to help with their recovery from the condition.

Postnatal depression also increased stress and created a wedge in the couples' relationships as men tried to cope with their partner's unpredictable moods. The partners spent longer at work or used alcohol to cope with women's depressive symptoms which resulted in less support to the women, and meant that women were often struggling with the bulk of child care and domestic duties. Supportive partners were those who listened to women's concerns, took days or weeks off work to provide practical assistance at home or nurtured women when they were depressed.

In the next chapter, we will explore the resolution of PND from women and their partners' perspectives.

References

Andreason, A., & Andreason, B. (1990). Toward a substantive theory of mother-twin attachment. *American Journal of Maternal Child Nursing, 15*, 373–377.

Areias, M. E., Kumar, R., Barros, H., & Figueiredo, E. (1996). Correlates of postnatal depression in mothers and fathers. *The British Journal of Psychiatry, 169*(1), 36–41.

Beck, C. T. (1996). Postpartum depressed mothers' experiences interacting with their children. *Nursing Research, 45*, 98–104.

Berggren-Clive, K. (1998). Out of the darkness and into the light: Women's experiences with depression of childbirth. *Canadian Journal of Community Mental Health, 17*, 103–120.

Boyce, P. (1994). *Use and misuse of the Edinburgh postnatal depression scale.* London: Gaskell.

Boyce, P. M. (2003). Risk factors for postnatal depression: A review and risk factors in Australian populations. *Archives of Women's Mental Health, 6*(Suppl. 2), s43–s50.

Brown, S., Lumley, J., Small, R., & Astbury, J. (1994). *Missing voices. The experience of motherhood.* Melbourne: Oxford University Press.

Buist, A., Barnett, B., Milgrom, J., Pope, S., Condon, J. T., Ellwood, D. A., et al. (2002). To screen or not to screen: That is the question in perinatal depression. *The Medical Journal of Australia, 177*(7 October), S101–S105.

Buist, A., Morse, C., & Durkin, S. (2003). Men's adjustment to fatherhood: Implications for obstetric health care. *Journal of Obstetric, Gynecologic, and Neonatal Nursing, 32*, 172–180.

Buultjens, M., & Liamputtong, P. (2007). When giving life starts to take the life out of you: Women's experiences of depression after childbirth. *Midwifery, 23*, 77–91.

Champion, L. A., & Goodall, G. M. (1994). Social support and mental health: Positive and negative aspects. In D. Tantum & M. Birchwood (Eds.), *Seminars in psychology and the social sciences.* London: Gaskell.

Chan, S., & Levy, V. (2004). Postnatal depression: A qualitative study of the experiences of a group of Hong-Kong Chinese women. *Journal of Clinical Nursing, 13*, 120123.

Cochran, S., & Rabinowitz, F. E. (2003). Gender-sensitive recommendations for assessment and treatment of depression in men. *Professional Psychology: Research and Practice, 34*(2), 132–140.

Condon, J. T., Boyce, P. M., & Corkindale, C. (2004). The first time father's study: A prospective study of the mental health and wellbeing of men during the transition to parenthood. *The Australian and New Zealand Journal of Psychiatry, 38*, 56–64.

Cox, J. L. (2005). Postnatal depression in fathers. *The Lancet, 366*, 982.

Currid, T. J. (2005). Psychological issues surrounding paternal perinatal mental health. *Nursing Times, 101*, 40–42.

Davey, S., Dziurawiec, S., & O'Brien-Malone, A. (2006). Men's voices: Postnatal depression from the perspective of male partners. *Qualitative Health Research, 16*(2), 206–220.

Dennis, C. L., & Ross, L. (2005). Relationships among infant sleep patterns, maternal fatigue, and development of depressive symptomatology. *Birth, 32*(3), 187–193.

Fettling, L. (2002). *Postnatal depression. A practical guide for Australian families*. Melbourne: IP Communications.

Fletcher, R. J., Matthey, S., & Marley, C. G. (2006). Addressing depression and anxiety among new fathers. *The Medical Journal of Australia, 185*(8), 461–463.

George, M. (1996). Postnatal depression, relationships and men. *Mental Health Nursing, 16*(6), 12–15.

Goodman, J. H. (2004). Paternal postpartum depression, its relationship to maternal postpartum depression, and implications for family health. *Journal of Advanced Nursing, 45*(1), 26–35.

Grant, B. (1995). Comorbidity between DSM-IV drug use disorders and major depression: Results of a national survey of adults. *Journal of Substance Abuse, 7*, 481–497.

Holopainen, D. (2002). The experience of seeking help for postnatal depression. *Journal of Advanced Nursing, 19*(3), 39–44.

Jeglic, E. L., Pepper, C. M., Ryabchenko, K. A., Griffith, J. W., Miller, A. B., & Johnson, M. D. (2005). A caregiving model of coping with a partner's depression. *Family Relations, 54*, 37–45.

Kitzinger, S. (1992). *Ourselves as mothers. The universal experience of motherhood*. London: Doubleday.

Kowalski, J., & Roberts, A. (2000). Postnatal depression: Involving partners in promoting recovery. *Professional Care of Mother and Child, 10*(3), 65–67.

Madsen, S. A., & Juhl, T. (2007). Paternal depression in the postnatal period assessed with traditional and male depression scales. *Journal of Men's Health & Gender, 4*(1), 26–31.

Matthey, S., Barnett, B., Ungerer, J., & Waters, B. (2000). Paternal and maternal depressed mood during the transition to parenthood. *Journal of Affective Disorders, 60*, 75–85.

Matthey, S., Barnett, B., Kavanagh, D. J., & Howie, P. (2001). Validation of the Edinburgh postnatal depression scale for men, and comparison of item endorsement with their partners. *Journal of Affective Disorders, 64*, 175–184.

Matthey, S., Barnett, B., Howie, P., & Kavanagh, D. (2003). Diagnosing postpartum depression in mothers and fathers: Whatever happened to anxiety? *Journal of Affective Disorders, 74*, 139–147.

Matthey, S., Kavanagh, D. J., Howie, P., Barnett, B., & Charles, M. (2004). Prevention of postnatal distress or depression: An evaluation of an intervention at preparation for parenthood classes. *Journal of Affective Disorders, 79*(1–3), 113–126.

Mauthner, N. S. (2002). *The darkest days of my life. Stories of postpartum depression*. Cambridge: Harvard University Press.

Meighan, M., Davis, M. W., Thomas, S., & Droppleman, P. G. (1999). Living with postpartum depression: The father's experience. *American Journal of Maternal Child Nursing, 24*(4), 202–208.

Milgrom, J., Martin, P. R., & Negri, L. M. (1999). *Treating postnatal depression. A psychological approach for health care practitioners*. Chichester: Wiley.

Misri, S., Kostaras, X., Fox, D., & Kostaras, D. (2000). The impact of partner support in the treatment of postpartum depression. *Canadian Journal of Psychiatry, 45*, 554–558.

Morgan, M., Matthey, S., Barnett, B., & Richardson, C. (1997). A group program for postnatally distressed women and their partners. *Journal of Advanced Nursing, 26*, 913–920.

Morrow, M., Smith, J., Lai, Y., & Jaswal, S. (2008). Shifting landscapes: Immigrant women and post partum depression. *Health Care for Women International, 29*(6), 593–617.

Morse, C., Buist, A., & Durkin, S. (2001). First-time parenthood. Influences on pre and postnatal adjustment in fathers and mothers. *Journal of Psychosomatic Obstetrics and Gynaecology, 21*, 109–120.

Nahas, V. L., Hillege, S., & Amasheh, N. (1999). International exchange. Postpartum depression: The lived experiences of Middle Eastern migrant women in Australia. *Journal of Nurse-Midwifery, 44*(1), 65–74.

O'Hara, M. W., & Swain, A. M. (1996). Rates and risk of postpartum depression: A meta-analysis. *International Review of Psychiatry, 8*, 37–54.

Paulson, J. F. (2010). Focusing on depression in expectant and new fathers. Prenatal and postpartum depression, not limited to mothers. *Psychiatric Times, 27*(2), 48–52.

Ramchandani, P., Stein, A., Evans, J., & O'Connor, T. G. (2005). Paternal depression in the postnatal period and child development: A prospective population study. *Lancet, 365*, 2201–2205.

Wilkinson, R. B., & Mulcahy, R. (2010). Attachment and interpersonal relationships in postnatal depression. *Journal of Reproductive and Infant Psychology, 28*(3), 252–265.

Wood, A. F., Thomas, S. P., Droppleman, P. G., & Meighan, M. (1997). The downward spiral of postpartum depression. *Maternal-Child Nursing Journal, 22*, 308–317.

Zelkowitz, P., & Milet, T. H. (1997). Stress and support as related to postpartum paternal mental health and perceptions of the infant. *Infant Mental Health Journal, 18*, 424–435.

Zelkowitz, P., & Milet, T. H. (2001). The course of postpartum psychiatric disorders in women and their partners. *The Journal of Nervous and Mental Disease, 189*, 575–582.

Chapter 8
Journeys to Resolution

Don't stay home, surround yourself with happy people and experiences, go to a group it's a good healing process [and] make yourself join things- have an outlet outside the home so you are not just a mother. You need an interest (Kris).

I would ring anyone, everywhere, whoever I could- I needed information. I always looked for help. I needed help and I looked for it- I didn't sit on my own and think about how bad it was. I needed people to help me; I needed to feel better about it (Erin).

The quotes given by Kris and Erin presented above reflect their journeys to resolution. In the previous chapter, we noted that only three women attributed hormonal changes to the onset of PND. The majority of women perceived that the lack of support from others contributed to their depressive symptoms and added to their feeling of isolation. Women's drawings captured the feeling that women were trapped, alone in the dark when they were diagnosed with PND.

The support from others was crucial in the process of resolution as it instilled hope that women could overcome PND. In our study, what was important was the quality of women's relationships with others, even one other person, on their journey to resolution. The following quote by Nicolson (1990: 693) highlights the importance of support in the postpartum period to prevent depressive symptoms:

The degree and quality of support in the early months of mothering was probably the single most crucial factor accounting for emotional stability.

The main focus of this chapter is the type of support women accessed when they were depressed, and the women's and their partners' perceptions of the efficacy of different biopsychosocial treatments for PND. This will be followed by a discussion of the barriers to accessing support. Finally, we will close with a discussion of women's experiences of reaching resolution where they felt comfortable with themselves as mothers and in their relationships with others. 'Resolution' seems a more appropriate term than 'recovery' as it implies that there has been a journey that shapes the individual, and can result in personal growth. Women's journeys to resolution will incorporate women's drawings and statements to provide rich accounts of their lived experience, and will also include the partners' perspectives.

C. Westall and P. Liamputtong, *Motherhood and Postnatal Depression: Narratives of Women and Their Partners*, DOI 10.1007/978-94-007-1694-0_8,
© Springer Science+Business Media B.V. 2011

8.1 Journeys to Resolution

Women received a range of treatments for PND including antidepressant medication or complementary therapies, plus either group and/or individual counselling. A large number of women reported feeling depressed for at least 2 years (range 3 months to 8 years). This finding is consistent with the American Psychiatric Association (2000) who claimed that 5–10% of the population may continue to have major depression for 2 years or more. In our study, some women experienced multiple episodes of PND (range one to three episodes), and two women relapsed within 2 years of their initial diagnosis. These findings are similar to Austin and Lumley (2003), who claimed that the recurrence rate of PND is 20–40% for Australian women. The high recurrence rate reflects the need for a biopsychosocial approach and an individual approach when treating women with PND.

Most of the women and their partners expressed the need for an individual approach when treating PND – an approach that was tailored to meet their individual needs. For example, treatment that focused on resolving women's individual triggers was more effective than the 'one size fits all' approach. Ned highlighted this point and also expressed the need for an individual approach when treating PND:

> I think all the combination that was put together to give her postnatal depression- triggered it - gradually those things that triggered it disappeared… It makes sense.

What worked for one participant did not work for another participant because of the tangled web of issues beginning for many women before the birth. What was evident from the women's stories is that they did seek help as they were all diagnosed with PND. Buist and colleagues (2005) suggested that women with PND sought help from family (50%), partner (29%), GP (29.2%) and maternal and child health nurse (28%), mainly for infant crying (40%), general advice (31%), not coping (30%) and sleep problems for themselves (19%) or their babies (17%).

8.2 Treatments

Most women were diagnosed with PND by a general practitioner, and the majority of these women were prescribed antidepressant medication. The predominant use of antidepressants to treat PND is also evident in the literature (Appleby et al. 1997; Beyond Blue 2006). Of interest, half of the women in our study who were prescribed antidepressants continued to be taking medication at the time of interview. Many of these women were still struggling with the concept of weaning off antidepressants when interviewed. The following quotes by Nicky and Katie highlight this dilemma:

> I tried to wean myself [off antidepressants] going back about three months ago, and ended up in a heap again. And I feel really good so I don't know why I regressed so much… They want me to go back in January and we'll try again. Maybe go down a little bit more gradually. Because I don't feel now that I have any issues or anything that I need to work through (Nicky).

I was weaned off the antidepressants very gradually, very slowly, and for the first few months being off the medication I was watching my emotions because I was really concerned in a way that perhaps I could relapse (Katie).

8.2.1   Antidepressants

Couples had mixed feelings about the use of antidepressant medication. Some participants refused to go on antidepressants, whereas others reached a point in their depression where they wanted a 'quick fix'. In general, women and their partners perceived that general practitioners and psychiatrists could have provided more information about the benefits and risks of antidepressant medication to be able to make an informed decision. As a result, couples expressed feeling disappointed and confused when they were making the choice about antidepressants. These findings are supported by Holopainen (2002), Mauthner (2002) and Steen (1996). Steen (1996) claimed that the lack of information about antidepressants resulted in feelings of anger, frustration and fear of the unknown. William, like many of the participants, was confused and concerned about the long-term use, addiction and changes to his partner's personality as a result of antidepressant medication:

At the start you've got no idea how long you're going to need to be on them [antidepressants]. You might only be on them for one month, two months, three months, but she [partner] is saying, "What happens if I'm not? I'm going to be on them for the rest of my life. How am I going to cope with my kids? Am I going to think the same way? Am I going to work things out the same way because I'm on this medication?"

Nicky too remarked that:

I'm not sure if it's an imbalance, a chemical imbalance now. I wish you could have that tested- a chemical test done so that there is something tangible and physical there. "Yes you have got that imbalance, and you're justified to feel the way you are, and be on the medication".

As previously discussed, researchers have identified the importance of educating women, not their partners. However, William's quote above highlights the need for couples to be educated about antidepressant medication. Whitton and associates (1996: 75) recommend that education of women is needed to improve the 'understanding and acceptance' of treatments:

Given that women are reluctant to accept drug treatment for their symptoms, ante-natal education may also improve women's understanding and acceptance of available treatments.

Women were also concerned about the long-term effects of antidepressant medication and feared addiction. In our study, most women took months or years to decide to take antidepressants, eventually succumbing to medication when they were in crisis. Other researchers have also suggested that women are reluctant to take antidepressant medication to treat PND (Appleby et al. 1997; Buist et al. 2005; McIntosh 1993; Whitton et al. 1996). McIntosh (1993) claimed that women took antidepressants as a last resort and when they had difficulty functioning. One participant in our study, Samantha, feared addiction and long-term dependency with antidepressant medication. After struggling with her symptoms of PND for 5 years, she wanted a 'quick fix' as she did not have the time to attend counselling or groups. When Samantha was asked what helped to relieve her depressive symptoms, she stated:

> The drugs, I needed a quick fix. I didn't need counselling or coming to group sessions. I didn't want to spend the time… It took me all of those years, five and a half years, to realise that maybe I had a problem [and] to take that step to do something about it. I had this mental negativity associated with drugs. Not that I associated with drugs, not that I labeled someone as on them…it's more I'm so afraid I'll get addicted to them and then I'll be on them the rest of my life, and then they'll have to keep upping the dose.

Unlike Samantha wanting the 'quick fix', for many participants, antidepressants were the last option as they preferred other treatments. Kris described antidepressants as the 'last option' to try when other treatments were unsuccessful:

> I saw that [antidepressants] as an absolute last option and I didn't feel like I was near that point. I felt that trying to do a course, or go to the gym and do things with people if that failed then okay. I just think drugs are handed out too easily these days and that you're not coping with it or dealing with it you're getting something to deal with it for you. I just think we're a society [where] we're just so quick to diagnose people with depression, 'Oh here's some drugs to pick you up', and that can create other problems… It scared me to go on drugs.

Many of the women and their partners feared addiction to antidepressants as they claimed they had addictive personalities or witnessed family members taking antidepressants for years. As previously discussed, many of the mothers of women were diagnosed with depression and PND. One participant claimed that her mother was taking antidepressant medication for 30 years. Danni was the only participant whose mother committed suicide. She feared taking antidepressant medication because her mother died of a pill overdose:

> I wouldn't take the antidepressants, flat out refused to take them. There's a family history of [taking] antidepressants. Pills have always scared me because mum died from a pill overdose. I would much rather have gone and had some counselling, seen a psychologist.

Women commonly voiced the need for someone to listen to them. Georgia needed someone to listen to her and to give her some solution or respite from motherhood:

> I probably didn't particularly want to go on antidepressants, but I felt if someone actually helped me with some of the very real barriers that I was facing I would be able to pull free [pause] because what I primarily was asking for help for was for A. [someone to] listen, and B. [someone to] give me some solution or respite from the enormity of mothering a baby that never stopped crying, and never slept, and that was probably what I wanted help with at that point.

Although women's views of PND differed from health professionals, most women reported a noticeable improvement in their mood several weeks after the initiation of treatment. When Marcia was taking antidepressant medication, she felt like she was moving 'out of this hole' and away from the darkness of her depression. She thought that her PND must have been partly biological as she felt an improvement in her mood 3 weeks after beginning treatment with antidepressants:

> Within three weeks [after starting antidepressants] I think I felt that I was clambering out of this hole I'd been in, and this cloud had lifted. I certainly felt a lot better than I did. So then to me it was proof that yes, there really was something wrong because I felt my mood and demeanor, and everything was so much better.

Most of the partners also noticed a reduction in the symptoms of PND as a result of antidepressant medication. Tim noticed his wife was more calm and rational, and was less anxious as a result of taking antidepressant medication:

> Once she started taking the antidepressants, after six or seven weeks you could certainly see the difference then- the anxiety level dropped, and she was a lot calmer and more rational about things.

Several men also noticed personality changes in their partner as a result of taking antidepressant medication. Some of these changes included a numbing of emotions and the reduced ability to deal with stress. Ned described antidepressants as the 'necessary evil'. He discussed how his wife became sedated and addicted to video games as a result of taking antidepressant medication:

> I could see a lot of secondary problems that came up as a result of her being on antidepressants but it's like a necessary evil… With the antidepressants she got really addicted to the most mind-numbing boring games that are on the computer and would just play them non-stop… That may have just been her way of coping until she was ready to come back to what she had to do… That really caused a lot of trouble between us.

As previously discussed in Chapter 4, the loss of libido was a particular concern for several women as it affected their intimacy with their partner.

Kristina was the only participant who was concerned with her memory loss after taking Zoloft. Although memory loss is also a symptom of depression, Kristina felt that her loss of memory was associated with taking antidepressant medication as she noticed a partial improvement in her memory when she came off antidepressants:

> The thing that plays on my mind now, even now is the memory loss associated with them [Zoloft]… When I came off [the medication] I got a bit of my memory back.

Kristina's husband, William, discussed her loss of memory as a significant change with antidepressants:

> To be honest her memory is a shadow of what it was. Just simple things- she couldn't tell you what she did five minutes ago at times…she gets very frustrated with that… Today that still adds to her lack of confidence, because she's not as confident as she used to be.

Women who were breastfeeding wanted to be informed about the effect of antidepressant medication on their babies. Tara wanted to avoid taking antidepressants as she was concerned about the long-term effects on the baby:

> I didn't get medication because I was very against it because I was being very careful about breast feeding… When I looked into antidepressants there are no long-term studies about the effect on the child… No-one could say to me, "Yes, these are safe". Some people would say, "Yes, these are safe", and then when I questioned them they actually re-stated it when they realised that I was going to ask questions. "They're not proven to be unsafe". Well that's very different to being safe.

Kath was concerned about her sedated infant when she breastfed her 10-month-old baby for the first time after taking the antidepressant, Cipramil. She was the only participant who weaned her baby because of the effect of the antidepressant medication. Kath reflected back on her experience:

> She [GP] just said, "you have got postnatal depression, and take the pills" and she wanted me to continue breastfeeding... But the first breastfeed I gave him after I took an antidepressant I just didn't like the look of him. He was just a very floppy baby that day and I said, "I'm not doing this to him. It's not fair". I stopped [breast]feeding after that.

Despite the widespread use of antidepressants, there has been little research investigating the efficacy of this form of medication (Cooper and Murray 1997; Hendrick 2003; Hoffbrand et al. 2006). Buist (2001) argues for depression to be treated aggressively with antidepressants even if the mother is breastfeeding to lessen depressive symptoms and to reduce the risk of psychosis. From a different standpoint, in the Cochrane Database of Systematic Reviews, Hoffbrand and colleagues (2006) caution the use of antidepressants in lactating mothers as there were no studies that identified the long-term effects on the infant. Studies that have examined the effects of antidepressant medication on breastfed infants have included healthy, full-term infants who are more likely to breakdown antidepressant medication than premature or sick infants (Wisner et al. 2002). Wisner and associates (2002) suggest that breastfeeding mothers are prescribed half the recommended dose of any antidepressant for 4 days only which can then be gradually increased until women's depressive symptoms are relieved. In the literature, there is evidence that babies can become sedated with antidepressant medication (Wisner et al. 1998, 1996). Buist (2001) advises health professionals to monitor babies closely for weight loss, sedation and developmental delay when breastfeeding mothers are taking antidepressant medication.

In a systematic review of the literature, Hoffbrand and others (2006) located only one trial that compared antidepressant medication with other forms of treatment. This trial by Appleby and colleagues (1997) revealed that fluoxetine (Prozac), a selective serotonin reuptake inhibitor (SSRI), was, after an initial session of counselling, as effective as a full course of cognitive behavioural therapy for treating PND. Following their review, Hoffbrand et al. (2006) argued that more trials are needed to compare antidepressant medication with psychosocial interventions and to assess the adverse effects of antidepressants. Holopainen (2002) claimed that further research is needed to determine women's perceptions of the efficacy of counselling and medication in the treatment for PND.

8.2.2 Electroconvulsive Therapy

Only one woman, Beatrice, received electroconvulsive therapy (ECT) to treat her PND. Electroconvulsive therapy is used when antidepressants are ineffective or when patients are psychotic (Victorian Drug Usage Advisory Committee 2003). The average course of ECT is six to ten treatments over 2–3 weeks, and the response rate for severely depressed patients is 50–80%, which is twice as effective as antidepressant medication (Victorian Drug Usage Advisory Committee 2003). However, controversy exists in the use of ECT as it induces a seizure in individuals. Research has not determined if it is the seizure itself or the chemical changes in the brain occurring after the seizure that relieves depressive symptoms (Block and Singh 1997). In our study, Beatrice was immune to a range of antidepressants and Lithium (a mood stabiliser). As a last resort, Beatrice received 12 sessions of ECT. Following these treatments, Beatrice knew she had to change her negative thinking to overcome her depressive symptoms and to avoid suicide:

> I'd tried so many different antidepressants and I seemed to be really quite immune to all of them, they had awful side effects. I tried everything and in the end I tried Lithium and that didn't do anything either. In the end he said the only other gun we've got really is shock treatment... They could do everything they could to me and none of it was making any difference. I know when I was depressed I was really angry a lot of the time, I was angry with Ethan [son]. But I think after the shock treatment perhaps because I knew that was the very last thing I knew it was either that or suicide. I must have just decided you've got two ways to go with this you've tried everything now there isn't anything else, you can either stay depressed, kill yourself or somehow make this enormous mental shift and decide that well he's difficult but that's your lot... I had to really stand behind my kid and be his advocate for him and that made a huge shift like suddenly it didn't matter.

8.2.3 Complementary Therapies

Some women used complementary therapies including Chinese herbs, acupuncture, naturopathic treatments, homeopathic remedies, yoga, Reiki and meditation. As with the antidepressants, women had mixed feelings about the benefit of these treatments. In general, women benefited from these treatments, as what worked for one woman did not work for another, possibly due to their level of depression at the time. Mary benefited from using acupuncture and Chinese herbs:

> I was seeing this Chinese acupuncturist and he had Chinese herbal medicines and that helped me to sleep properly and I really felt good while I was doing that. I feel like that really finished off the whole process.... I went to a healer as well- that was while I was on medication and doing the group therapy- and that just involved Reiki and aromatherapy.

Tara also did Reiki and took evening primrose oil:

> [I tried] the evening primrose oil which regulates your hormones a bit. I had done Reiki before... I think it did help to relax me at times. I think that helped a bit.

Melissa tried aromatherapy:

> I've always been into aromatherapy a little bit, so I paid more attention to which oils actually had antidepressant qualities and things like that, but I didn't use them as an alternative. I stuck with the antidepressants, but on days when I was particularly depressed, or feeling a bit low, I actually used the appropriate oils.

Barbara discussed the benefit of yoga:

> The one thing my doctor made me do was going and doing yoga... and I loved it, it was just absolutely brilliant, the thing for me... I haven't done it for over a year, and I'm missing it dreadfully. My state of mind is probably not as even as it was when I was doing it... I always found the relaxation before and after hard, but I slept better when I came home, it just helped me so [emphasised] much (Barbara).

Tessa found that naturopathic treatments were helpful:

> I've got a close relationship to my naturopath and if I needed to I would have gone to tell
> my GP but at that stage I thought I'd try the natural remedies first... She said that I had a
> chemical imbalance in the brain and she put me on vitamins B5's and B6's and I called them
> my happy drugs! I probably had a sixty to seventy percent improvement once those kicked
> in- within a few days I felt so much better. So that was a huge shift.

Erin tried naturopathic and homeopathic treatments:

> I went to see this naturopath, because I thought, "I don't want to do this [PND] again", and
> I told him that. He said to me that he believed that postnatal depression... or maybe it was
> isolated to postnatal, was [due to] a big drop in magnesium. He believed it was hormonal,
> and I do believe that because a couple of weeks ago... he gave me magnesium, zinc and
> calcium, and homeopathic drops and homeopathic pills for my anxiety. **And those helped
> with the anxiety?** Oh definitely.

In contrast to Erin and Tessa, Sue was more depressed when she took naturopathic treatments. This could have been due to her level of depression at the time:

> My friend, her parents were... naturopaths. They were like you come over here we're going
> to cure you of your depression; we're going to get you out of your depression without
> Prozac. I went over there with extremely high expectations of they think they can cure me...
> It didn't work and I left there more depressed. They tried herbs, they tried diet, they tried
> acupuncture and nothing helped. They were also helping me with my weight because that
> was another depression factor, I was 50 pounds heavier than I had ever been in my entire
> life and that was depressing for me. I left worse off.

Erin benefited from meditation:

> I'd done a lot of work on myself on a spiritual level, and I work well that way, so for me
> meditation helped me a lot- doing the time out, and doing the breathing.

Unlike Erin, Danni found that meditation was ineffective:

> I got back into my meditation [but] you can't meditate when you're depressed it's impossible
> to meditate when you're in that depression.

8.2.4   Individual Counselling and Cognitive Behavioural Therapy

Most women expressed the need for individual counselling to relieve their depressive symptoms. Similar findings have been reported in the literature (Beck 1993; Buist et al. 2005; McIntosh 1993; Priest et al. 2006). Researchers have identified that resolving past difficulties can resolve PND (Berggren-Clive 1998; Mauthner 2002; Nicolson 1999). Mauthner (2002) pointed out that women who resolved past issues and conflicts were more content with their roles as mothers. Nicolson (1999) suggested that women gained strength and competence when their past difficulties were managed appropriately. Not surprisingly, Nicolson (1999) revealed that poor mental health was associated with unresolved difficulties surrounding loss. In our study, some of the issues that women needed to have addressed were related to childhood sexual abuse, blended families and relationship difficulties, particularly issues with their own mothers. Mary expressed the benefit of having individual counselling to discuss issues with her mother, as well as group counselling, to reduce the isolation associated with PND:

> I think it's really a combination of a lot of things. I don't think any one thing can work on its own. I really believe you've got to have a combination of the medication, counselling and relaxation techniques... I still had issues with my mum that weren't being resolved so that was a constant thing holding me back from getting me better.

Katie expressed her desperate need to talk to someone when she was depressed:

> I had to have regular visits to the GP and they would assess me every time. But the GP- as lovely as the GP was- didn't actually suggest any counselling, they just gave me the medication. Looking back now I can remember thinking counselling would have been good because your mind is in such a mess really, you really have a need to speak to somebody and talk to them about these problems that you have. I remember thinking, "Why does no-one want to ask me what's really the matter and what's upsetting me?"

Tara told us that individual counselling was helpful:

> Individual counselling- that's what I really needed. That person could have said to me, 'A lot of people feel that way'. I did need some one on one in-depth, "Why did you feel that way about that? Why do you think you're not a good mother?" I needed more of that, and once I got more of that I did start improving.

Some couples benefited from couple's counselling, as Sarah mentioned:

> After Kevin's breakdown it's been so much easier, we've done a bit of counselling together which is something he said 'never'. Yeah it's been much better.

Cognitive behavioural therapy helped to lower women's expectations of themselves. In Berggren-Clive's study (1998), women with PND felt a lift in their depression when they adjusted their unrealistic expectations of themselves. Val found that cognitive behavioural therapy challenged her expectations of herself and her children, and this helped her to resolve her depressive symptoms:

> [The psychiatrist said], "you know this is what you're expecting to be... perfection. You can't be there. You can strive for there but you'll never get there"... so learning to be a bit kinder to myself [and] learning to be a bit kinder to my kids.

Telephone support lines were an affordable service that offered individual counselling and they could remain anonymous. The benefit of telephone support was that women could access this support most of the time and in the privacy of their own homes. This type of support was invaluable to women who wanted to talk to a health professional who understood PND. As Kim remarked:

> When I rang XXXX they were very helpful because the girl had been through it, she knew what it was like and she could pre-empt some of what I was going to say.

8.2.5 Support Groups

Most women who were recruited into the study attended postnatal support groups facilitated by a maternal and child health nurse or a psychologist to resolve their PND. These groups enabled women to talk about PND with other women who experienced the condition and gave women the opportunity to be honest about how they were feeling. Groups were particularly beneficial for women with insufficient support as it gave them the opportunity to talk about their experience of motherhood and PND. Almost all of the women who attended support groups reported a lift in their depression when their feelings were validated by others in the group, and they benefited from the comfort of knowing that they were no longer alone in their misery. Kelly, like many other women who attended a support group, maintained lasting friendships with other group members. She felt that others in the group were not judgmental and could understand her situation:

> Having others to talk to was the biggest thing for me, because I didn't have anyone to talk to. [My partner] was [saying], "Get on with it. Get over it. Move on". It was good to be able to talk about [PND] and knowing you're not the only one… I felt like no-one judged me and thought how stupid I was for not having a natural birth.

Katie also realised she was not alone when she attended the group, and it forced her to get out of the house:

> Going to the support group I realised that I wasn't alone and [pause] there were other people that were going through the same thing as me so it did really help. It [group] was something to break up your week because with postnatal depression I felt at times very isolated because your confidence takes a real nose-dive and when you do meet people I felt personally I had nothing to contribute to the conversation. I felt like you know who would want to speak to me? So you really tend to stay home more with that condition. So the support group actually helped to get me out of the house and meeting other people, and helped me to realise that I wasn't a failure- it was a condition and the condition would go away eventually. That really helped.

Similarly, Monica thought that her feelings were validated when she attended the support group. She also benefited from feeling like others understood her situation and offered support:

> I can tell you to this day the best [emphasised] thing I did was the [support] group. That was the first time I felt validated. It was the first time I met with a group of people that didn't judge me. That was the best thing [laughs]. Had I not done anything else I still would have done that. It was the first time that he [baby] had screamed his head off, and people came and comforted me rather than trying to comfort him, that was the big change for me. I had so many people say to me, "I've been where you're at". No-one had said that before.

Lyn also told us that the support group was the most helpful treatment:

> I think we're all on the same level and we all never overpowered each other and it was wonderful. It was the best thing I ever did.

Kim benefited from talking to others who experienced PND as it helped her to understand the condition:

> I guess the reassurance that other people have gone through this, and… hearing other people's stories really helps you understand it [PND].

Support groups also provided an opportunity for women to share their feelings about motherhood. Bridget and Nancy wanted to speak to women who felt the same way about motherhood:

> Meeting the other person in the group, I really clicked with [her]. We were both on the same wave length as to how we actually felt about motherhood… [She] can actually understand that it's hard work rather than just joy (Bridget).

> It was really good to be in a very small group with women that didn't feel like being jolly, but just wanted to talk about anything or share their experiences, and have a bitch about it or get angry about it, and that seemed more real to me (Nancy).

Beatrice found attending the group motivated her to do things:

> For that hour or hour and a half a week you'd have to throw it all out on the table and face it for a while and own up to it. Perhaps in the process of making suggestions to other people, everyone was suggesting have you tried this, what about trying that, that you actually start healing yourself a little bit too, by pooling all your own resources. Because in theory you're pooling that with someone else but why they're at it you think I might actually do that too.

Support groups also gave women hope and strength to conquer the bad days and an awareness that PND would pass over time. The notion of hope from attending support groups for women with PND has been reported in previous studies. Berggren-Clive (1998) suggested that support groups created hope for women as they realised they were not alone. Similarly, Beck (1993) argued that support groups instilled hope that women could resolve their depressive symptoms and be in control of their lives. When Denise attended the support group, she gained hope that future episodes of PND were 'just a short emotional feeling':

> There is light at the end of the tunnel. If in the future we [support group] have to go down that path again, you know it's just a short emotional feeling.

Although sharing experiences of PND was helpful for some women, only three women who attended support groups did not benefit from this type of support as they wanted to move away from talking about PND. For these women, there was a fine line between talking to others and women wanting to escape from talking about PND. Holopainen (2002) has also argued similarly that women who attended support groups were unable to take anyone else's problems on board. Kristina and Denise expressed the difficulty being around other depressed people as it lowered their mood:

> I was having a good day. I felt being around all the other people who were obviously not having good days I felt like I was dragged down. That's a really important thing…for everyone to understand from day one that they may go backwards and it's actually scary…you feel like you're losing the plot again, it's very frightening (Denise).

Researchers have identified the benefit of support groups to reduce depressive symptoms in women (Beck 1993; Berggren-Clive 1998; Buultjens et al. 2008; Holopainen 2002; Scattolon and Stoppard 1999; Steen 1996; Tomison 1999). Similar to the findings from our study, Holopainen (2002) argued that women who attended support groups felt less isolated, made lasting friendships with others and felt understood and accepted. Buultjens and colleagues (2008) evaluated a holistic support group that ten Australian women with PND attended. Buultjens et al. (2008) revealed that holistic support groups improved the mother–infant bond and reduced maternal anxiety levels, and concluded that this type of support group could be used by midwives, maternal and child health nurses and other trained health professionals.

8.2.6   Respite in Early Parenting Centres and Mother–Baby Units

Almost half of the women required admission to a mother–baby unit or residential early parenting centre for respite, treatment and help with sleep routines to improve their emotional well-being. Women also compared themselves with other mothers. In general, most women benefited from this type of support as they received a combination of treatments and were able to have some respite from motherhood. They also received assistance with difficulties relating to infant sleep and settling problems, and their emotional well-being was also assessed and monitored. Denise, Val and Erin discussed the support they received in the mother–baby unit:

> I had three weeks [in the mother-baby unit] and had my meals brought in, all I had to think about was getting better. Another thing too, we did yoga and the cognitive thinking with the psychiatric nurse [in the mother-baby unit]. If anything I personally felt that was the biggest [help], medication aside, because actually it's all in here again [points to head]. It's actually how you talk to yourself (Denise).

> [In the mother baby unit] I was seeing him [the psychiatrist] for probably two hours a week, and to be able to talk about stuff, even think about it, talk it over with Noah, and one of the nurses. I found that really valuable to be able to go over that with people who understood and had some kind of background with it, plus some experience that was really quite valuable. I really learnt a lot about myself in there. It saved me [pause], it saved my kids too… When you get up instead of thinking about all the things you've got to do that day, thinking about the three things that you're really happy about today (Val).

> When I went into the mother-baby unit we were both patients- we didn't know whether it was her or whether it was me, and they sort of treated her for colic or reflux. So they were giving her Mylanta…but she was beautifully settled in there, because my whole energy and demeanor had changed- I felt more confident, I learnt skills to be a mother (Erin).

Danni and Sarah remarked about early parenting centres:

> The fact that they [early parenting centre] weaned him was huge, absolutely huge because I stopped looking at him as a parasite because I felt like he was just feeding, living off me. Once I stopped breastfeeding that gave me a bit of a chance to get some weight back on… we did baby massage, we had nice groups with nice soft meditation music, baby massage, groups where staff would take the children and the mums would have time out. At home he was on the bottle which meant dad could feed him. One of the nurses at [early parenting centre] gave me a fantastic piece of advice and it was don't give into him, the first time you do that's it, you're back at the beginning (Danni).

> It [early parenting centre] was the most amazing place. The fact they told me, "look, she [baby] is okay. We can fix this". But also it was like a hotel, I had my own room, they brought me food all the time and Debra came to visit and there was somewhere to play. It was fantastic, two of the best days of my life! It was just such a relief (Sarah).

Several women, like Marcia, were unable to continue the sleep strategies when they got home:

[After being in the early parenting centre], I just couldn't [continue the strategies]- he broke me in the end. We did weeks of controlled crying, and in the end I succumbed, and he ended up back in our bed again- just sanity to get sleep.

But for some women, like Beatrice, they found that their admission created more stress:

I used to walk the corridor in tears. I think because they [early parenting centre] keep the babies in the nursery obviously so you can sleep, so they can look at their patterns and have a go at taming them. Then being separated from her just caused a big melt down, I was in floods of tears continuously. I could hear her crying and I would walk up and down look through the glass [and] that was really killing me. I did have a meltdown while I was there.

Researchers have examined the benefit of psychosocial treatments in the resolution of depressive symptoms (Appleby et al. 1997; Holden et al.1989). In an intervention study of newly delivered mothers, Holden and colleagues (1989) claimed that women who received non-directive counselling from health visitors showed a significant improvement in mood. The health visitors were given a short training course in counselling techniques. Appleby and others (1997) compared pharmacological and psychological interventions to determine the optimal treatment for non-psychotic depression. The psychological intervention included counselling based on cognitive behavioural therapy. Women were randomly allocated to one of four intervention groups, each woman received a combination of fluoxetine or placebo, and either one session or six sessions of counselling. The individual counselling sessions enabled women to talk about their circumstances, experiences and feelings, and aimed at exploring four areas: negative beliefs, current circumstances, childcare/time management and relationship with partner. The counselling was given by a research psychologist under the supervision of a psychiatrist. Appleby et al. (1997) concluded that provided the reluctance of women to accept pharmacological treatment, counselling services need to be more readily available for women suffering from PND.

In a systematic review of the literature, Dennis and Creedy (2006) assessed the effects of psychosocial and psychological interventions before, during and after the birth to reduce the risk of PND. They examined 15 trials involving over 7,600 women and identified that diverse psychosocial and psychological interventions failed to reduce the number of women who developed PND. The psychosocial interventions included antenatal and postnatal classes, professional continuity of care and early postpartum follow-up. The psychological interventions included debriefing and interpersonal psychotherapy. These interventions were provided by physicians, nurses and midwives. Dennis and Creedy (2006) contend that the only intervention that would potentially reduce PND was intensive, professionally based postpartum support provided by health professionals.

In the Cochrane Database of Systematic Reviews, Ray and Hodnett (2006) examined studies that used professional and/or social support interventions for PND including emotional support, counselling, tangible assistance and information delivered by telephone, home or clinic visits, or individual or group sessions, compared with any form of usual care for depressed mothers. Ray and Hodnett (2006) located only two studies (Appleby et al. 1997; Holden et al. 1989) and a total of 137 women that compared additional support from caregivers with usual forms of care in the postpartum period. These women were clinically depressed within six months after the birth. Ray and Hodnett (2006) found that the common outcome for both trials was a reduced level of depression at 25 weeks postpartum, which was significantly lower in the groups receiving additional support.

8.2.7 *Interpersonal Support*

When interpersonal support was provided, it was beneficial to women's emotional well-being because it provided women with the opportunity for respite and to talk about their feelings. This type of support included accepting help, exercise, returning to work and spiritual support (church groups, prayer). The support the partners provided was discussed in Chapter 4. In general, women felt a lift in their depressive symptoms when they received practical support (assistance with childcare and household chores), when they received emotional support (the feeling of being understood by others, particularly their partners) and had time for themselves.

Most women were unable to tell their family and friends about their PND until they were on the journey to recovery. They feared that no-one could possibly understand how they were feeling. In her research, Mauthner (2002) claimed that partners, families and friends were not significant in the recovery process as women could not access this support until they were on the road to recovery. In Mauthner's (2002: 157) study, one woman stated: 'I couldn't talk to family and friends until I was at a certain point in recovery', and another: 'In the depths of depression, I didn't want to talk to a soul about it. I just didn't think there was any point'. Similarly, Holopainen (2002) contended that families were often unaware of the mother's condition as they were frequently unable to tell them about their problems. In our study, Kim was unable to talk with her friends about her depression as she perceived herself as a failure. When she was on the road to recovery, she was able to talk with them openly about her depression:

> Initially, I just didn't want them [friends] to see that I had failed, that I was so miserable... It wasn't until I was on the road to recovery that I could talk to them about it [PND].

Once women accepted practical help, they appreciated the assistance of others:

> Accepting help when it was offered even if it was someone coming around and sitting here, and I'd go for a walk. Just getting out into the outside world for half an hour on your own. It was so important to have that time on your own with your own thoughts whether it be a bath, go for a walk, read a book. Really that was just sacred to me (Ellie).

> My girlfriend came over and she would come and she'd vac the floor- she wouldn't ask she'd just go to my cupboard and do it. But she's that type of person (Kristina).

I had a lot of support with getting meals prepared, I've got two older sisters... and my mother's group as well were supplying my meals, so I could get all my washing done (Erin).

I just couldn't get the housework done, so I employed a cleaner to come once a fortnight, and she still comes (Marcia).

Exercise was beneficial for some women:

Carolyn: You said going to the gym was important in your recovery as well?
Tessa: Yes, absolutely partly because it was part of my old lifestyle, and partly because the feel good side of it, just feeling good about yourself and also getting your body [laughs] back to some sort of normality. I'm lucky in that the gym I go to has got a really good child care centre where I don't have to rely on anyone else.

Katie suggested similarly:

I've really kept active- I enjoy power walking when I can... just having other things to focus on has really been helpful.

Most women who returned to work perceived that it helped to reduce their depressive symptoms as it provided them with the opportunity to increase their social network and to rejoin the community. Kim discussed how returning to work helped in the recovery process as she enjoyed working:

[My daughter] was five and a half months when I returned to work and that helped with my recovery. Yes, going back to work for me was a real goal because I enjoyed my job, I loved my job and I had never not worked.

Similarly, Beatrice found that returning to work helped with the resolution of her depressive symptoms as she escaped from the domestic realm of motherhood and rejoined the wider community:

Working was really good. Putting [the children] into crèche was really important. I'd go and have lunch with a friend or sit down and finish something I was making, go for a swim. I always tried to do something with that time. Sometimes I would just sleep if I was really ragged but I wouldn't just sit and read the paper I would actually do something, that was pretty important. Yes, any of those things you did outside of your domestic motherhood realm that were creative or somehow out in the wider community, or just for yourself they were very useful.

Although women generally benefited from returning to work, it created additional stress and was a juggling act, as Denise stated: 'Going back to work was quite frightening. It was another stress'. Elisabeth and Georgia remarked as follows:

I didn't like the work it was causing fights because I didn't like leaving Kane, so I ended up resigning after about ten weeks. I just wasn't happy (Elisabeth).

I was going to work, and at times I'd have to stop the car because I was passing out from tiredness, and you know I was in a tremendously responsible job at that time (Georgia).

The tension between balancing paid work with unpaid work associated with motherhood has also been reported by Hoschschild (1997).

Spiritual support assisted some women with their depressive symptoms. Three women thought that their faith in God helped to resolve their depressive symptoms. In Nims's research (1996), women with PND reported a spiritual component to their recovery. Spiritual support is an important aspect of support (Nasser and Overholser

2005). Spiritual beliefs can provide hope and promote recovery from depression (Braam et al. 1997). In our study, Katie and Diane felt that their faith in God helped to resolve their depressive symptoms and instilled hope:

> I think just having my faith helped to get through it a lot too... Just having that hope there has just made a real difference to me (Katie).

> I'm Christian so I find that God really helped me as well (Diane).

Over the past two decades, the spiritual component has been added to Engel's (1977) biopsychosocial model to form the biopsychosocial–spiritual model (Carson and Arnold 1996). The spiritual dimension encompasses an individual's spiritual beliefs as an important component of their health and provides a more holistic approach to health care. However, the definition of spirituality can be limited to a Christian view of religion (Nooney and Woodrum 2002; Stolley et al. 1999) rather than a broader concept of spirituality (Gall et al. 2005). Spirituality can also provide hope and optimism when individuals experience suffering (Schwab and Petersen 1990). The spiritual self is based on individual moral values and beliefs as they strive for meaning in their everyday lives (Carson and Arnold 1996).

Researchers have identified the importance of support to assist women's recovery from PND (Brown et al. 1994; Holopainen 2002; Mauthner 2002; Ugarriza 2002). In a Victorian longitudinal study, Brown and colleagues (1994) interviewed women when their babies were 8–9 months of age and again when their children were 2 years of age. In Brown et al.'s (1994) study, the most common reason women felt their emotional well-being improved was related to their child getting older (52%), having more support from their partners (31%), going back to work (27%) and not feeling so tired (25%). Of major significance was the fact that less than 4% of women stated that professional intervention (either counselling or medication) was a major factor in their recovery. Ugarriza (2002) claimed that over half the women in her study who were diagnosed with PND needed time away from the baby and the overwhelming responsibility of motherhood to be able to recover from PND. However, the partners' perspectives are missing from these studies.

8.2.8 Barriers to Accessing Support

The barriers to accessing support fell into two categories – internal and external barriers. when support was difficult to access, partners, family members, friends and neighbours were instrumental in convincing women that they needed professional help.

8.2.8.1 Internal Barriers

Most women were aware of the support services available. However, the internal barriers to getting help included women not wanting to burden others, perceptions of themselves as 'bad mothers', financial difficulties and the lack of private health insurance. Many women discussed the difficulty in tapping into their support networks as they did not want to burden or worry others or did not want to be rejected if they asked for help. In general, women wanted people to offer support, rather than having to ask for it. The burden was related to others being busy with their own lives. In their study, Harrison and colleagues (1995) argued similarly that the barriers to getting support were reluctance to ask for support, lack of reciprocity, perception that the use of support would burden others and non-supportive messages included within supportive actions. In our study, the following quotes highlight the difficulty women had tapping into their support networks:

> That was my fault for not reaching out to people. I wouldn't call my mum in England for years, I'd only ring her and pretend everything was wonderful. I don't want to upset her (Sarah).

> I haven't had as much support down here as in friendships and that sort of thing because everyone's got other things happening in their lives, and I don't want to be a burden to other people- my own worst enemy! (Kath).

> The first time I didn't tell anyone, the second time I didn't really tell anyone so it's hard to get support if you don't tell anyone (Val).

A major barrier to getting help for their depressive symptoms was women's fear that they would be labelled as 'bad mothers'. Despite frequent visits to the maternal and child health nurse in her child's first year, Val, a third-time mother with a history of undiagnosed PND with her first two children, was scared to admit that she was unable to cope with the pressure of motherhood:

> I knew all the places I could go to get help I just didn't… It's not in my nature to admit that I'm not coping… If you've never failed anything to then fail at the one thing that is supposed to be natural and normal and everyone else is doing it, and everyone else appears to be doing a great job. It's hard to say, 'I can't do this'.

Tara also had difficulty tapping into her support network after the birth. Unlike Val, Tara became depressed so quickly that she was unable to access the practical and emotional support she needed:

> I remember it [PND] was mentioned in the antenatal classes and I think we were given… some of the signs you may experience, and the partners were there for that as well. I had suffered depression before so I know what those signs are. And she [nurse] did talk about having structures in place. [She said], "You need to think ahead about who you would call on if you're having a hard time, and have some practical support as well as emotional support"… I think I just became so insular so quickly that I wasn't able to see those things and I wasn't able to access them anyway.

Financial difficulties and the lack of private health insurance were two other barriers to getting treatment. The cost of ongoing psychiatric visits and counselling sessions deterred many women from accessing this type of support. For some women, the lack of private health insurance meant they could not access the support they needed in mother–baby units and instead had to go on lengthy waiting lists to early parenting centres. Holopainen (2002) has pointed out that the lack of private health insurance was a barrier to getting treatment in Australia. In our study, some women had difficulty accessing support from health professionals as they were not privately insured:

> We'd spent a lot [emphasised] of money on counselling, and we don't have private health cover so it was an awful drain financially. The financial problems led to more stress. We spent a lot of money on solicitors and psychologists and really achieved not a great deal (Marcia).

> She's a private psychiatrist- it's a hundred and ten dollars you've got to find to pay beforehand. We're on a safety net now so we get it back but it's just the hassle of going to Medicare after you've been there… [and] finding someone to look after two kids (Kath).

8.2.8.2 External Barriers

For most women, the major external barriers to accessing support were the failure of health professionals to identify women's symptoms of PND and the lack of awareness of support services. This meant they continued to struggle with their depressive symptoms without the professional intervention they desperately needed. Many of the health professionals ignored women's desperate cries for help or were unable to help women when they had difficulties with feeding and settling their infants. Similarly, Wood and colleagues (1997) argued that women's concerns about the baby were ignored by health professionals. Bridget's maternal and child health nurse ignored her cries for help when she developed symptoms of PND. When she was asked what advice was unhelpful, she replied:

> I reckon that initial advice saying that it [PND] is normal [from the maternal and child health centre]… just saying, 'You're sleep deprived and it's normal to be feeling the way you are'.

Similar sentiments were expressed by Ellie:

> My doctor dismissed me [when he said], "You're just going through a tough time, it will get better"… He didn't give me the reaction I wanted. He said to me, "do you have any thoughts of hurting yourself or your baby?" And I said, "no, never"… He said, "Well, you're alright. Babies get older and get easier", and sent me on my merry way. I said to him, "I cry every day, it's just not what I thought it would be, it's so much harder. This baby just cries; I don't feel like I've bonded with her".

The health professionals also had difficulty labelling women's experiences as PND. This quote also shows the health professional's lack of understanding about PND and the fact that women could talk themselves into depression. Perhaps this is why women received insufficient information about PND from some health professionals. Katie's quote highlights this dilemma:

> I went off to the GP and they realised there was something wrong too. I think from memory I didn't straight away go onto the medication- they said, "Oh you don't want to talk yourself into postnatal depression. Let's see how you go". And anyway I didn't go very well. So I returned to the doctors and said, "I'm not coping".

Georgia was disappointed that her maternal and child health nurse was unable to provide assistance with settling her baby. She discussed the lack of support she experienced after the birth of her first child:

> I went and saw the [maternal and child health] nurse there, and I remember telling her how I felt, and how my baby wasn't sleeping, and she basically turned around and told me to "pull up my socks", and she was absolutely god awful. I have since heard similar things [laughs]. She basically told me to, "get a grip". And she said, "you just need to do such and such"… I just thought this is who it seemed logical for me to go and talk to!

Denise, a third-time mother, considered the general practitioner to be unhelpful when she refused to check her thyroid level as she would be reprimanded for over-servicing. There is evidence that thyroid dysfunction can cause depression (Cohen 2007). Denise was later diagnosed with the condition Hashimoto's thyroiditis when she was admitted to a mother–baby unit:

> The GP didn't help …that's where she didn't pick it up [thyroid problem]. She didn't want to do the blood test again because I had one six weeks ago, because she thought she would be wrapped over the knuckles for over-servicing.

Pregnant women and women contemplating future pregnancies discussed the need to seek out supportive health professionals if they developed PND again. These women voiced the need to access professional help earlier if depressive symptoms developed with their next baby. Ellie, a first-time mother, wanted to avoid her previous maternal and child health nurse as she was not receptive to PND:

> Next time around I'll change [maternal and child] health nurses [quiet voice] to someone who's a bit more receptive to people, to postnatal depression.

Monica was six months pregnant and discussed the need to get a referral to the psychiatrist in case she developed depressive symptoms after the birth:

> We've had a few little things happen with this pregnancy… I was straight down to my GP, and said, "This is happening, and I'm really quite concerned that I can see that depression creeping in, and I don't want to go there again. I don't want that. Can you keep an eye on me?"… I guess I'm really aware of it, and probably a bit paranoid [laughs] about ending up there again. I've got a referral letter sitting on the fridge for a psychiatrist to even go and meet prior to this baby being born so that I've got a relationship with someone in case things happen again.

The failure of health professionals to identify PND has been reported by other researchers (see Holopainen 2002; Mauthner 1993, 2002; McIntosh 1993; Meighan et al. 1999; Whitton et al. 1996; Wood et al. 1997). Wood and associates (1997) claimed that women with PND perceived the health professionals as unhelpful when they were unable to understand women's experiences and normalised their symptoms of depression. Mauthner (1993, 2002) found that when women disclosed their depression to health professionals, they did not always get the understanding and support they needed. McIntosh (1993) contended that health visitors dismissed women's feelings of depression as normal and offered no other assistance or advice.

Whitton and colleagues (1996) argued that 29% of health visitors normalised women's symptoms of depression as they believed it was normal to feel anxious or miserable when caring for a baby. Following a training session, only 8% of health visitors held this belief, highlighting the need to educate health professionals.

The lack of support from health professionals when women are diagnosed with PND has been reported in numerous studies (Beck 1996; Dennis 2003; Holopainen 2002; Mauthner 1993, 2002; Morrow et al. 2008; McIntosh 1993; Meighan et al. 1999; Nicolson 1990; Wood et al. 1997). McIntosh (1993) suggested that the lack of support from health visitors and general practitioners in acknowledging women's feelings meant that these mothers were not assisted to treatment or offered support groups because they did not believe these women were depressed. Similarly, Dennis (2003) compared the perceived helpfulness of health services among depressive and non-depressive women and found that depressed women were more likely to rate the health professional as unhelpful when they failed to address their health issues. Mauthner (2002) argued that women felt less depressed when they were able to talk about their feelings in a non-judgmental environment.

Researchers have identified that women's views of PND differed from the medical perspective of PND (Buist et al. 2005; McIntosh 1993; Morrow et al. 2008; Priest et al. 2006). Buist and others (2005) revealed that women preferred psychological and social management rather than drugs for PND. McIntosh (1993) contends that women's perceptions of their problems were not treatable with antidepressants. Morrow and associates (2008) found that some women benefited from antidepressant medication, but women viewed PND as a psychosocial problem.

8.3 Women's Experiences and Drawings of Resolution

Some qualitative studies have explored the resolution of PND from women's perspectives (Berggren-Clive 1998; Holopainen 2002; Mauthner 1995, 1998, 1999, 2002; McIntosh 1993; Nicolson 1990, 1999; Nims 1996). However, these studies concentrated on women's experiences, and the men's experiences were incidental findings (Condon et al. 2004). Furthermore, no visual representations of resolution for women with PND were found in the literature.

In our study, the final stage of resolution occurred when women accessed support from others. There was no easy transition to resolution for these women. As previously discussed, women struggled to access support from others, struggled to get the right treatment for their depression and struggled to come to terms with the illness. Some women described this stage as a 'turning point' where they accessed support from others, and over time felt a lift in their depressive symptoms. Resolution also occurred when women paid more attention to meeting their needs and adjusted their expectations of others. The process of resolution resulted in women feeling emotionally well, hopeful about the future and content in their relationships, particularly with their partner and children. In contrast to the biomedical understanding of PND, most women preferred resolving underlying psychosocial issues that contributed to their depressive symptoms. Resolution also incorporated the feeling of hope that women could cope with the bad days and any further recurrences of PND. Accessing support was an important part of women's resolution from PND. Similar findings were documented by Mauthner (2002) and Berggren-Clive (1998). Berggren-Clive (1998) claimed that women resolved PND when they surrendered (accessed help), were hopeful (received support) and rebuilt their sense of self (adjusted their expectations and met their own needs).

The resolution from depression has been defined as a period of eight consecutive weeks with no more than one or two mild depressive symptoms (Keller et al. 1987). Similar to findings by Berggren-Clive (1998), the shift from depression to resolution among the participants in our study was not linear. Instead, the pathway to resolution was a process of having ups and downs, or good weeks and bad weeks, making it difficult for women to know when PND finally ended. As one partner in the focus group, Nathan, stated: 'There's no line that says, 'you're over it''. Women's drawings and verbal accounts showed a shift from darkness to light and colour; however, remnants of darkness remained in most of the drawings representing the bad days, and not PND.

8.3.1 From Darkness to Light and Colour

All of the women's drawings of resolution portrayed bright colours and were instilled with hope. In their verbal accounts, they described resolution in terms of a lifting of the darkness they experienced when they were depressed towards the light that represented resolution. In their retrospective accounts of PND, women described PND as 'a passing cloud', 'the occasional black cloud that drifts across still', 'there are still clouds on the side', 'the cloud would be nearby' and 'there is still a dark cloud, but it has lifted'. Other women spoke about resolution as a lifting fog instead of a cloud. Sometimes, resolution was described as a physical transition up a mountain, or away from the isolation of a bucket, tunnel, hole or forest that represented depression, to a place where they were supported by others.

Women's drawings are not about the success of antidepressants, but about how a combined approach led to the resolution of the women's PND. No drawings were located that showed a visual portrayal of resolution. This was evident as only one woman placed a health professional into her drawing of PND. Women's drawings of resolution were filled with hope and stood in stark contrast to their drawings of PND. These visual images showed a dramatic shift away from depression. Most drawings of resolution showed a small area of darkness. The darkness represented the bad days that were an inevitable part of life, but through their experience of PND, women gained strength and a sense of hope that they were prepared for these bad days. The feeling of hope occurred when women gained strength knowing they could overcome the bad days or any further episodes of PND. Women also gained hope when they felt supported by others. Hope is a cognitive construct that requires motivation and goal-directed behaviour (Snyder et al. 2003). Resolution was also a

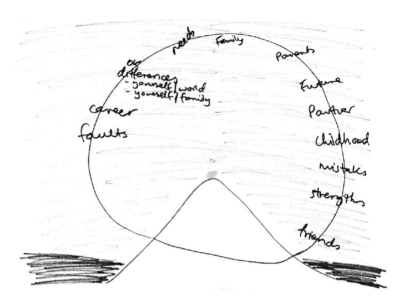

Fig. 8.1 Beatrice's image of resolution

time where women realised they were no longer alone and had reconnected with others, including their partners and babies.

Beatrice, a mother of two, was the only participant who struggled with PND for 8 years. She was diagnosed with PND during her first pregnancy and was treated with antidepressants, mood stabilisers and ECT. At the time of interview, she was no longer taking antidepressant medication. She described resolution as a physical lifting up a mountain above the quagmire that represented her depression below. On top of the mountain, she was able to have a clear perspective of relationships, needs, issues and the future. Resolution represented 'lightness, goodness [and] positive things'. When Beatrice was asked to describe her drawing (Fig. 8.1), she stated:

> I've drawn a mountain only in the sense that I wanted to convey a feeling of having really risen up something. What I've drawn below that mountain is black; it's the black lagoon I suppose. The sense of me being the little bright yellow dot has risen above that black mire to a point where you get a perspective. The blue I've drawn all around is that feeling of perspective, yes, that there's a panorama. That you're not actually caught in a black tunnel looking through a pin hole of light, you are actually way, way out in that light. The yellow is lightness, goodness [and] positive things.

Beatrice's drawing (Fig. 8.1) shows a physical move away from her depression, represented by the darkness, or 'quagmire' as she described it. At a point of resolution she had risen up a mountain to have a clear perspective of life. When she was depressed, she was unable to identify her needs or goals.

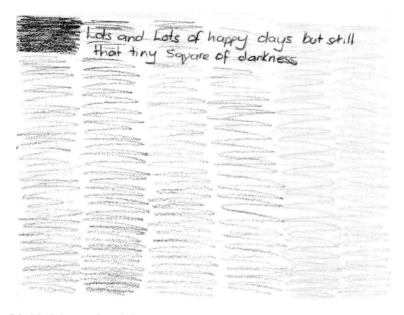

Fig. 8.2 Meg's image of resolution

8.3.2   Remnants of Darkness

Most women's drawings of resolution showed remnants of darkness, which is a normal part of life. The darkness that remained in these drawings was unrelated to the duration or severity of PND, or antidepressant use. As with Beatrice's image of resolution, for most women, resolution represented light and colour with a small area of darkness that represented their bad days. Like many female participants, Meg's image of resolution (Fig. 8.2) stands in stark contrast to her drawing of PND as total darkness in the previous chapter (Fig. 6.1) as it shows both light and colour. Meg was diagnosed with PND when her baby was 7 weeks old. She stated that her PND lasted for '1–2 months' even though she was still on medication at the time of interview when her baby was 11 months old. Meg described her drawing of resolution (Fig. 8.2) as 'Lots and lots of happy days, but still that tiny square of darkness'. Meg gained strength and a sense of hope that she was prepared for the bad days she was experiencing. When Meg was asked how she was feeling then compared with the darkness, she replied:

> Towards the end of it but you can never guarantee that you're not going to have a bad day but they don't last forever like it did back at the start. I can go for a month without having a bad day. Now I see colour and light, now 6 days or 7 days out of 7 are nice. If you had to draw a picture now what would it look like? It would have colour this time. Nice happy colours- a bit of red, not as much black, I think I'd only draw one square black instead of the whole page… It's still in the back of your mind, it's not 100 percent gone but you can deal with it. So instead of being just pitch black it might be charcoal [laughs].

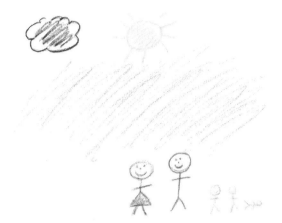

Fig. 8.3 Marcia's drawing of resolution

Similar to Meg's drawing, Marcia's drawing of resolution also showed a small area of darkness (Fig. 8.3). Marcia, mother of three children, was diagnosed with PND when her second baby was 8 weeks old. Her PND lasted for 18 months and was treated with antidepressants. At the time of interview, she was no longer taking antidepressant medication. Marcia's darkness in her image of resolution represented a 'few days that aren't always happy'. When she was asked to describe her drawing of resolution, she replied:

> Now there's happiness, and I feel supported, and [there is] me as a family. There's still a dark cloud but it's lifted. Obviously there are a few days that aren't always happy, but that's where I'm at.

In contrast to Meg and Marcia's images showing small areas of darkness, Kristina and Sue's drawings of resolution showed no evidence of darkness. Kristina's drawing of resolution (Fig. 8.4) portrayed a happy, bright image, compared with her image of PND in the previous chapter (Fig. 6.3). Kristina was diagnosed with PND immediately after her first child's birth and 1 month after her second baby's birth. Both episodes of PND lasted for 9 months and were treated with antidepressants. Kristina was no longer taking antidepressants at the time of interview. She described her drawing of resolution as 'happy and bright':

> It's bright… there's nothing not to be happy about. I'm back to being able to find the positive in everything no matter if something bad happens I'll still [put] the positive spin on it. Even when I was going through the depression I thought this is happening to me for a reason. I know good's going to come out of this, I don't know what it is, something good's going to come out of it…My bright, happy future now. Yes, I'm happy. Yes, loving life, and just living it up and having a great time. **There's no darkness in that picture?** [There is] absolutely none, none at all. When it's happy and bright I think of rainbows [laughs].

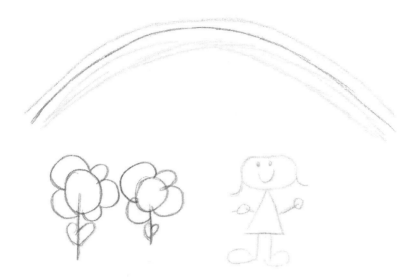

Fig. 8.4 Kristina's image of resolution

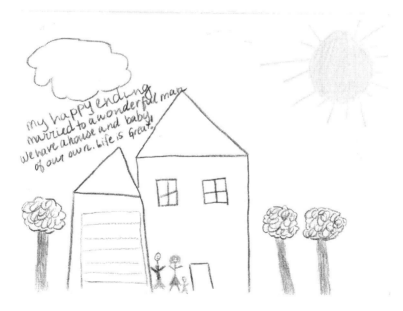

my happy ending
married to a wonderful man
we have a house and baby
of our own. Life is great.

Fig. 8.5 Sue's image of resolution

Sue's image of resolution also showed no evidence of darkness (Fig. 8.5). This image stood in stark contrast to her drawing of PND in the previous chapter (Fig. 6.8) where she planned her death by car exhaust. Her drawing of resolution was filled with hope for the future and enjoying her life with her husband and daughter. Sue was diagnosed with PND 4 weeks after her second birth when her baby was adopted out.

She was depressed for 3 years. Sue described her drawing of resolution as dreams from her childhood coming true:

> The next one is my happy ending, sun shining, blues skies, a few clouds, some trees, our house, my husband, which I need to draw some hair on him [laughs] and our daughter. All of my dreams have come true, I've got a wonderful husband- Christian man, we're involved in a good Church, [I am an] at-home mum. I've got my own baby. There's a lot of hope. We're looking at starting our family expansion in September, so we'll have another baby. It's just my whole dream from growing up…Now I've got my own house and husband and my own mum [mother in law] and it's like everything, all my dreams from my childhood have come true. It's like okay what's next because this is as far as my dream went so it's causing me to dream bigger and better. My business is taking off, I'm probably busier than I should be but I'm enjoying it [laughs]. It has been quite the journey, I'm just glad that I've been able to touch other people by my story and know that it can get better, it will get better, you've got to work through it, just don't end it.

Georgia's description of resolution also showed hope. Georgia was diagnosed with PND shortly after her first and second children's births and lasted for over 2 years. Georgia was not treated with antidepressant medication. Georgia's image of PND where she concisely stated 'I'm in a box, and I'm alone' (Fig. 6.4) also stood in stark contrast to her description of resolution that was far more descriptive:

> Motherhood is like life… a long, slow river. I have perhaps turned the bend and hopefully gone through the turbulent squall, but every day it continues to flow and turn with the wind. The journey is ongoing, but I can certainly smile and anticipate the challenges, though sometimes the here and now is hard.

Women's interviews were also filled with hope and highlight the notion that PND can be resolved. The following quotes illustrate this:

> We've gone through it again, listened to ourselves [and] listened to others… okay we're better now. We had gone down and back up again, good, there is light at the end of the tunnel. If in the future we have to go down that path again, you know it's just a short emotional feeling, because postnatal depression is such a constant thing you feel like you're never, ever going to get better (Denise).

> It's been a good thing for me in that I'm far more understanding of other people and I'm not as quick to judge them (Tessa).

> I feel good now… I feel like I've resolved all of the things that needed to be dealt with so I think that's a good place to be (Val).

> Looking back I think I've matured a lot through it all. I've probably grown a lot as a person. I guess I've really grown up I think. It's changed me- I'm probably not the same person I was beforehand, I feel like I've changed to a certain extent. But where I am now, I still feel like I'm growing, I'm really discovering who I am still but I'm starting to feel more content with life now… I've always felt perhaps there was a reason I went through this because I can help other people going through it. If ever there's people I know of or friends going through it at least I can relate now better with them, and I can have a greater understanding of it (Katie).

> It's like I've got power back in my life, and control back in my life. Now it's just working out putting me into the equation of what I want for me I suppose (Nicky).

> I just feel like I'm back to my normal self. And I just feel like Nerissa's at an age now like she's really good, she understands. She just talks to you like we talk, she's amazing. She's just so easy to look after- she's not so dependent on you… it does get easier and they're not so dependent (Margaret).

Having gone through that has made me stronger. Having gone through my mother's death has made me stronger, but at the time you feel like you're going to crumble. But when you're on the other side and you're looking back you think, "I've come so far, and have got so much strength from it" (Erin).

8.4   Chapter Summary

Most of the women and their partners expressed the need for an individual approach when treating PND designed to meet their individual needs. Women commonly voiced the need for someone to listen to them when they were diagnosed with PND. In general, women and their partners were concerned about the long-term effects of antidepressant medication and were concerned about the risk of addiction and personality changes associated with its use. Breastfeeding mothers were also concerned about the effects of antidepressants on their babies.

Many women were disappointed when health professionals dismissed their cries for help. As a result, the treatment and support that women needed were not offered to them. The barriers to accessing support included women's own fear of burdening others or being rejected by others if they asked for help. Financial barriers meant that women were limited in their treatment options. Many women found that health professionals had difficulty identifying the symptoms of PND and resulted in a late diagnosis of PND.

Women reported a lift in their PND when they accepted help and support from others, such as offers of respite, practical help or treatment for their depressive symptoms. The effectiveness of treatments depended on the individual and highlights the need for an individual approach when treating PND. Some women described resolution as a 'turning point' when they rejoined the community, felt emotionally well, had a clear perspective of life, were hopeful about the future and were happy with their relationships with others. Support groups provided the opportunity for women to meet other women experiencing PND and reduced the shame and isolation women were experiencing. Although women's drawings of resolution identified the physical shift away from PND, most drawings showed remnants of darkness that represented their bad days. In general, women's drawings of resolution were filled with light, colour and hope, and also showed the presence of others. Their drawings and stories highlight the notion that PND can be resolved.

References

American Psychiatric Association. (2000). *Diagnostic and statistical manual of mental disorders, text revision. DSM-IV-TR* (4th ed.). Washington, DC: American Psychiatric Press.

Appleby, L., Warner, R., Whitton, A., & Faragher, B. (1997). A controlled study of fluoxetine and cognitive-behavioural counselling in the treatment of postnatal depression. *British Medical Journal, 314*(7085), 932–936.

Austin, M. P., & Lumley, J. (2003). Antenatal screening for postnatal depression: A systematic review. *Acta Psychiatrica Scandinavica, 107*(1), 10–17.

Beck, C. T. (1993). Teetering on the edge: A substantive theory of postpartum depression. *Nursing Research, 42*, 42–48.

Beck, C. T. (1996). Postpartum depressed mothers' experiences interacting with their children. *Nursing Research, 45*, 98–104.

Berggren-Clive, K. (1998). Out of the darkness and into the light: Women's experiences with depression of childbirth. *Canadian Journal of Community Mental Health, 17*, 103–120.

Beyond Blue. (2006). What is postnatal depression? http://www.beyondblue.org.au/index.aspx?link_id=94. Accessed 12 June 2007.

Block, S., & Singh, B. S. (1997). *Understanding troubled minds. A guide to mental illness and its treatment.* Carlton South: Melbourne University Press.

Braam, A. W., Beekman, A. T., Deeg, D. J., Smith, J. H., & van Tilburg, W. (1997). Religiosity as a protective or prognostic factor of depression in later life: Results from a community survey in the Netherlands. *Acta Psychiatrica Scandinavica, 96*, 199–205.

Brown, S., Lumley, J., Small, R., & Astbury, J. (1994). *Missing voices. The experience of motherhood.* Melbourne: Oxford University Press.

Buist, A. (2001). Treating mental illness in lactating women. *Medscape Women's Health, 6*, 1–7.

Buist, A., Bilszta, J., Barnett, B., Milgrom, J., Erickson, J., Condon, J. T., et al. (2005). Recognition and management of perinatal depression in general practice. A survey of GP's and postnatal women. *Australian Family Physician, 34*(9), 787–790.

Buultjens, M., Robinson, P., & Liamputtong, P. (2008). A holistic programme for mothers with postnatal depression: Pilot study. *Journal of Advanced Nursing, 63*(2), 181–188.

Carson, V. B., & Arnold, E. N. (1996). *Mental health nursing. The nurse-patient journey.* Philadelphia: W.B. Saunders.

Cohen, A. (2007). Treatment of anergic depression in Hashimoto's thyroiditis with fluoxetine and D-amphetamine. The thyroid/depression connection. http://www.thyroid-info.com/articles/cohen.htm. Accessed 12 June 2007.

Condon, J. T., Boyce, P. M., & Corkindale, C. (2004). The first time father's study: A prospective study of the mental health and wellbeing of men during the transition to parenthood. *The Australian and New Zealand Journal of Psychiatry, 38*, 56–64.

Cooper, P., & Murray, L. (1997). Prediction, detection, and treatment of postnatal depression. *Archives of Disease in Childhood, 77*(2), 97–99.

Dennis, C. L. (2003). Influence of depressive symptomatology on maternal service utilization and general health. *Archives of Women's Mental Health, 7*, 183–191.

Dennis, C.-L., & Creedy, D.K. (2006). Psychosocial and psychological interventions for preventing postpartum depression. *Cochrane Database of Systematic Reviews, 1*.

Engel, G. L. (1977). The need for a new medical model: A challenge for biomedicine. *Science, 196*, 129–136.

Gall, T. L., Charbonneau, C., Clarke, N. L., Grant, K., Joseph, A., & Shouldice, L. (2005). Understanding the nature and role of spirituality in relation to coping and health: A conceptual framework. *Canadian Psychology, 46*(2), 88–104.

Harrison, M. J., Neufeld, A., & Kushner, K. (1995). Women in transition: Access and barriers to social support. *Journal of Advanced Nursing, 21*, 858–864.

Hendrick, V. (2003). Treatment of postnatal depression. *British Medical Journal, 327*(7422), 1003–1004.

Hoffbrand, S., Howard, L., & Crawley, H. (2006). Antidepressant treatment for post-natal depression. *Cochrane Database for Systematic Reviews, 1*, No page number.

Holden, J., Sagovsky, R., & Cox, J. L. (1989). Counselling in a general practice setting: Controlled study of health visitor intervention in the treatment of postnatal depression. *British Medical Journal, 298*, 223–226.

Holopainen, D. (2002). The experience of seeking help for postnatal depression. *Journal of Advanced Nursing, 19*(3), 39–44.

Hoschschild, A. (1997). *The time bind.* New York: Metropolitan Books.

Keller, M. B., Lavori, P. W., & Friedman, B. (1987). The longitudinal interval follow-up evaluation: A comprehensive method for assessing outcome in prospective longitudinal studies. *Archives of General Psychiatry, 44*, 540–548.

Mauthner, N. S. (1993). Towards a feminist understanding of 'postnatal depression'. *Feminism and Psychology, 3*(3), 350–355.

Mauthner, N. S. (1995). Postnatal depression: The significance of social contacts between mothers. *Women's Studies International Forum, 18*, 311–323.

Mauthner, N. S. (1998). It's a woman's cry for help: A relational perspective on postnatal depression. *Feminism and Psychology, 8*, 325–355.

Mauthner, N. S. (1999). "Feeling low and feeling really bad about feeling low": Women's experiences of motherhood and postpartum depression. *Canadian Psychology, 40*(2), 143–161.

Mauthner, N. S. (2002). *The darkest days of my life. Stories of postpartum depression.* Cambridge: Harvard University Press.

McIntosh, J. (1993). Postpartum depression: Women's help-seeking behaviour and perceptions of cause. *Journal of Advanced Nursing, 18*, 178–184.

Meighan, M., Davis, M. W., Thomas, S., & Droppleman, P. G. (1999). Living with postpartum depression: The father's experience. *American Journal of Maternal Child Nursing, 24*(4), 202–208.

Morrow, M., Smith, J., Lai, Y., & Jaswal, S. (2008). Shifting landscapes: Immigrant women and post partum depression. *Health Care for Women International, 29*(6), 593–617.

Nasser, E. H., & Overholser, J. C. (2005). Recovery from major depression: The role of support from family, friends, and spiritual beliefs. *Acta Psychiatrica Scandinavica, 111*, 125–132.

Nicolson, P. (1990). Understanding postnatal depression: A mother-centred approach. *Journal of Advanced Nursing, 15*, 689–695.

Nicolson, P. (1999). Loss, happiness and postpartum depression: The ultimate paradox. *Canadian Psychology, 40*(2), 162–178.

Nims, C. L. (1996). *Postpartum depression: The lived experience.* Unpublished Master's thesis. Medical College of Ohio, Toledo.

Nooney, J., & Woodrum, E. (2002). Religious coping and church-based social support as predictors of mental health: Testing a conceptual model. *Journal for the Scientific Study of Religion, 41*(2), 359–368.

Priest, S.R., Austin, M., & Sullivan, E.A. (2006). Antenatal psychosocial screening for prevention of antenatal and postnatal anxiety and depression. *Cochrane Database for Systematic Reviews, 1*, No page number.

Ray, K.L., & Hodnett, E. D. (2006). Caregiver support for postpartum depression. *Cochrane Database for Systematic Reviews, 1*, No page number.

Scattolon, W., & Stoppard, J. M. (1999). "Getting on with life": Women's experiences and ways of coping with depression. *Canadian Psychology, 40*(2), 205–219.

Schwab, R., & Petersen, K. U. (1990). Religiousness: Its relation to loneliness, neuroticism, and subjective well-being. *Journal for the Scientific Study of Religion, 30*(4), 381–394.

Snyder, C. R., Lopez, S. J., Shorey, H. S., Rand, K. L., & Feldman, D. B. (2003). Hope theory, measurements, and applications to school psychology. *School Psychology Quarterly, 18*(2), 122–139.

Steen, M. (1996). Essential structure and meaning of recovery from clinical depression for middle-adult women: A phenomenological study. *Issues in Mental Health Nursing, 17*, 73–92.

Stolley, J. M., Buckwalter, K. C., & Koenig, H. G. (1999). Prayer and religious coping for caregivers of persons with Alzheimer's disease and related disorders. *American Journal of Alzheimer's Disease, 14*(3), 181–191.

Tomison, A.M. (1999). *Creating the vision: Communities and connectedness.* Paper presented at the Child Expo, Melbourne, 22 April 1999.

Ugarriza, D. N. (2002). Postpartum depressed women's explanation of depression. *Journal of Nursing Scholarship, 34*(3), 227–233.

Victorian Drug Usage Advisory Committee. (2003). *Therapeutic guidelines: Psychotropic* (5th ed.). North Melbourne: BPA Print Group.

Whitton, A., Warner, R., & Appleby, L. (1996). The pathway to care in post-natal depression: Women's attitudes to post-natal depression and its treatment. *The British Journal of General Practice, 46*, 427–428.

Wisner, K. L., Perel, J. M., & Findling, R. L. (1996). Antidepressant treatment during breast-feeding. *The American Journal of Psychiatry, 153*(9), 1132–1137.

Wisner, K. L., Perel, J. M., & Blumer, J. (1998). Serum sertraline and N-desmethylsertraline levels in breast-feeding mother-infant pairs. *The American Journal of Psychiatry, 155*, 690–692.

Wisner, K. L., Parry, B. L., & Piontek, C. M. (2002). Postpartum depression. *The New England Journal of Medicine, 347*(3), 194–199.

Wood, A. F., Thomas, S. P., Droppleman, P. G., & Meighan, M. (1997). The downward spiral of postpartum depression. *Maternal-Child Nursing Journal, 22*, 308–317.

Chapter 9
Postscript

This book has explored the different pathways that couples perceived to have contributed to their emotional well-being. As previously discussed in this book, the emphasis was placed on the psychosocial aspect of the biopsychosocial model by identifying the importance of support before and after the birth. The partner's stories matched the women's narratives regarding the lack of support.

The findings from Chapters. 1–5 are presented in the following section, outlining the personal and professional support that women needed before and after the birth.

9.1 Couples Experiences of Parenting and PND

9.1.1 In Pregnancy and Childbirth

Most women were disappointed with the amount of support they received from health professionals in pregnancy and childbirth and resulted in the loss of self-esteem and sense of failure. The majority of couples discussed the scant amount of information about PND they received in antenatal classes to be able to understand the condition, and this resulted in difficulty identifying symptoms after the birth. The dramatic portrayal of PND in the media – where women killed themselves or their children – skewed their views of PND as they perceived it was a severe condition.

Some women expressed the need for counselling when they were faced with abnormal antenatal tests or experienced pregnancy losses, and this affected the attachment to their baby as they feared they would lose the baby. Most women perceived their childbirths were traumatic and reported negative perceptions of their childbirth experiences, and several women experienced post-traumatic stress disorder.

C. Westall and P. Liamputtong, *Motherhood and Postnatal Depression: Narratives of Women and Their Partners*, DOI 10.1007/978-94-007-1694-0_9,
© Springer Science+Business Media B.V. 2011

9.1.2   After the Birth

Most women in this study discussed the enormous challenges associated with motherhood and difficulty adjusting to their new role. Multiparous women had the added expectation of being perceived as experts. Societal myths about being a 'good mother' only disempowered women and contributed to their sense of personal failure. In hospital, women were disappointed with the conflicting advice they received from midwives about breastfeeding, and the lack of assistance with infant feeding and settling difficulties to reduce maternal sleep deprivation and fatigue in the postnatal period and to lessen anxiety. Many couples talked about the pressure to breastfeed and struggled with feelings of being a failure if they were experiencing difficulties. Most women were disappointed with the amount of support they received from health professionals, partners, friends and their own and other mothers after the birth for their emotional well-being. This resulted in the loss of self as a result of the multiple losses women perceived they experienced as mothers.

In the early postpartum period, most women described feeling different to other mothers before they were diagnosed with PND. The notion of feeling different to other mothers has not been documented in the literature prior to the onset of PND and is an important finding as it has implications for detecting early symptoms of PND.

9.1.3   Postnatal Depression

Women were often in crisis when they sought help for their depressive symptoms. Most couples were aware that there was something wrong when women developed symptoms of PND. Most couples identified that PND was caused by the stress associated with motherhood (Berggren-Clive 1998) rather than hormonal changes. Couples wanted to be informed about the range of treatments available and were concerned about the long-term effects of antidepressants and addiction.

Maternal sleep deprivation due to unsettled infant behaviour was identified by couples as the main trigger for PND. The partners were also struggling with the lack of sleep. Most women reported a delay in bonding to their babies when they were depressed, particularly when they had unsettled infants. These are early warning signs for PND. The ongoing sleep deprivation resulted in severe fatigue, exhaustion, social isolation and the loss of control. Women's visual portrayal of PND highlighted the themes of being trapped and alone in the dark and created feelings of helplessness and despair. Women commonly voiced the need to escape from the burden of childcare and household duties that represented motherhood.

Although most women in this study attended PND support groups, only three women did not benefit from this type of support. These support groups allowed women to talk about the challenges associated with motherhood and reduced their feelings of isolation. In general, most women voiced the need for individual counselling as it gave them the opportunity to discuss their individual issues related to childhood sexual abuse, grief and loss, blended families and relationship difficulties, particularly with their own mothers.

Most women expressed the need for someone to listen to them and for an individual approach when treating PND. Women's drawings of resolution identified the physical shift away from PND, but most drawings showed remnants of darkness that represented their bad days. In general, women's drawings of resolution were filled with light, colour and hope. Women's drawings and stories highlight the notion that PND can be resolved.

9.2 The Partners Experiences of PND and the Impact of PND on the Partner

The partners felt helpless and were unsure how to support women when they developed PND as they were excluded from treatment plans to be given strategies to support women and to understand the condition. Two partners were diagnosed with depression when women recovered, and two men with a history of depression noticed a worsening of symptoms when women recovered. The partners were the main source of support for women. However, most women were disappointed with the amount of support they received from their partners. The partners struggled to provide support because they had difficulty understanding PND as they were not included in treatment plans. Most of the couples felt that PND created a 'wedge', 'a wall' or 'barrier' in the couple's relationship.

9.3 Implications for Practice

There are many areas that need to be addressed in relation to clinical practice and policy development.

1. The number of women who were survivors of childhood sexual abuse, adult rape and domestic violence indicate a need for prenatal screening to identify women who may be particularly vulnerable to experiencing PND.
2. Health professionals caring for women in labour need to ensure that women have adequate pain relief and to be informed about the progress of their labours. They also need to ensure that women are provided with an opportunity to have debriefing after the birth to discuss their childbirth experiences and to reduce their sense of failure.
3. Parenting groups are needed to dispel the myths of motherhood, to educate couples about PND and to teach parenting skills. Ideally, these topics should

be discussed in antenatal classes rather than after the birth. With a better understanding about PND, couples would be able to observe for symptoms.

4. Health professionals need to listen to women's concerns and how they are coping with their baby. Women with unsettled infants need additional support from health professionals and possible referral to other support services.
5. Screening women with the EPDS in pregnancy and after the birth should be carried out, but women's scores may be higher than recorded. A clinical interview needs to follow any screening tool to identify women's individual needs and concerns and to diagnose PND.
6. Health professionals need to take women seriously and to listen to their concerns and assist them with their difficulties. If they are unable to assist women, they need to refer women to other services.
7. Including the partners in treatment plans when women are diagnosed with PND is crucial so that they can be given strategies for supporting women and to understand the condition.
8. Screening the partners for PND using the EPDS and using a clinical interview to confirm diagnosis, particularly when women recover from PND should be conducted.
9. Health professionals need to offer an individual and holistic approach to treatment rather than just offering antidepressant medication.

9.4   Specific Contributions of This Research

The findings from this study have increased the understanding and resolution of PND. Interviewing the partners added depth and dimension to women's stories and has contributed to the newly emerging field, where men are included in studies relating to PND. Women's drawings were a powerful portrayal of their experiences of PND and resolution. Many studies have explored the lived experience of PND. However, this study is unique as it included women who had resolved PND and their partners' perspectives. This study has identified that support is beneficial to women's mental health and has provided new insights into the psychosocial factors that affect women's emotional well-being.

The findings we have presented in this book could be used to inform and develop programs to identify women who are particularly vulnerable to experiencing PND, or to improve the treatment of the illness to assist other families in their recovery. The findings of this study will also enable health professionals to reflect on their existing understanding of PND and to understand the complex needs of women and their partners in pregnancy, childbirth and in the postpartum period. Families who are contemplating pregnancy, or parents themselves relate to some of the issues that have been discussed in this book and will hopefully gain additional support by reading this book.

9.5   Directions for Future Research

Important findings have emerged from the participants' stories. As with any qualitative study, the aim of our study was not to generalise to a wider population, but to explore how women and their partners understand and resolve PND. From this study, several important themes have emerged that warrant further investigation, such as: the feeling of being different to other mothers after the birth, the impact of maternal sleep deprivation on emotional well-being, escape and suicidal intent and the emotional well-being of partners, particularly when women resolved PND. Future research also needs to include different ethnic groups as they may experience PND differently to women in this study. Future research would also benefit from qualitative studies investigating different health professionals' experiences of women with PND, such as counsellors, doctors, midwives and maternal and child health nurses. It would also be beneficial for future research to include women who do not seek treatment for PND. Do they have a longer course of PND? How does their experience of PND differ? What factors are important in their recovery?

9.6   Conclusion

In conclusion, PND is a growing public health problem. Health care reform has done little to improve the emotional well-being of women after the birth. Early discharge from hospital has meant that women have less time to learn about mothering skills and to recover from the birth. Shrinking community services that focus on treatment and not prevention has added to the burden of PND in our society. As women are unlikely to identify their own symptoms of PND they need the support from others. Health professionals play a role in educating couples about PND, providing emotional support and identifying symptoms of PND. If health professionals dismiss women's cries for help, women and their partners may face months or years of misery, struggling to access the much needed support to set them on the path to resolution. Health professionals can also assist women with feeding and settling problems in the postpartum period to assist women in their adjustment to motherhood and to reduce their sense of failure. The challenge for health professionals also lies in women acknowledging their distress. Increasing the awareness of PND may help to reduce the stigma associated with PND so that women feel comfortable asking for help and to assist others in identifying women's symptoms.

The partners were the main avenue of support for women. However, the partners also need to be assessed for PND included in treatment plans and to be given strategies to support women. By caring for the partners as well as the women, health professionals can minimise the risks of cognitive, emotional and behavioural problems on children and improve family functioning.

Reference

Berggren-Clive, K. (1998). Out of the darkness and into the light: Women's experiences with depression of childbirth. *Canadian Journal of Community Mental Health, 17,* 103–120.

Appendix A: Glossary of Terms

Antenatal/antepartum	Pregnancy
Foetal death in utero	The loss of a pregnancy after 20 weeks gestation
Gestation	Pregnancy
Infanticide	The act of killing an infant
In utero	In pregnancy
Miscarriage	The loss of a pregnancy before 20 weeks gestation
Multipara/multiparous	Women with more than one child
Perinatal	The period shortly before and after the birth
Prenatal	Pregnancy
Postnatal/postpartum	After the birth
Primipara/primiparous	Women with one child
Puerperium	Up to 6 weeks after the birth

C. Westall and P. Liamputtong, *Motherhood and Postnatal Depression: Narratives of Women and Their Partners*, DOI 10.1007/978-94-007-1694-0,
© Springer Science+Business Media B.V. 2011

Appendix B: Demographics of Participants

Female Participants

Interview	Pseudonym	Age	Occupation	Children	Diagnosis of PND	Age at diagnosis
1	Mary	39	Secretary	3	1999	34
2	Meg	25	Childcare	1	2004	25
3	Sue	29	Own business	3	1999	24
4	Kim	30	Nurse	1	2004	30
5	Beatrice	43	Student	2	1989	38
6	Danni	43	Rep	1	1992	31
7	Elisabeth	33	Home duties	3	2001	30
8	Kelly	34	Phone operator	3	2001	31
9	Bridget	36	Receptionist	2	2001	33
10	Denise	40	Medical rep	2	2001	37
11	Samantha	36	Sales	2	2002	34
12	Kris	38	Fashion design	2	2001	35
13	Tessa	39	Music teacher	2	2003	38
14	Sarah	39	Administrator	2	2001	36
15	Lyn	36	Office worker	3	2001	33
16	Val	35	Teacher	3	2002	33
17	Nancy	41	IT consultant	2	2003	40
18	Katie	39	Dental nurse	2	2001	36
19	Kath	32	Nurse	2	2003	31
20	Ursula	29	Insurance	2	2002	27
21	Nicky	34	Teacher	3	2002	32
22	Monica	32	Engineer	1	2002	30
23	Kristina	35	Rep	2	2002	33
24	Georgia	36	Assistant mgr	2	2002	34
25	Marcia	36	Nurse	3	2002	34
26	Maria	29	Nurse	2	2001	27

(continued)

Female Participants (continued)

Interview	Pseudonym	Age	Occupation	Children	Diagnosis of PND	Age at diagnosis
27	Margaret	34	Secretary	1	2002	32
28	Ellie	32	Stock control	1	2003	31
29	Erin	30	Legal secretary	1	2002	28
30	Melissa	33	Aromatherapy	2	2002	31
31	Diane	27	Doctor	1	2005	27
32	Barbara	43	House duties	3	1997	35
33	Tara	34	Teacher	1	2003	32

Male Participants

Interview	Pseudonym	Age	Occupation	Depression
1	Shane	48	Transport	No
2	Neil	42	Accountant	No
3	Noah	36	Owner driver	No
4	Kevin	41	Data cabler	Yes
5	Ned	40	Sales/ IT	No
6	Liam	31	Engineer	No
7	Kyle	59	Nurse	Yes
8	Tim	37	Carpenter	No
9	Luke	33	Engineer	No
10	William	43	Fleet manager	No
11	Robert	35	Sales manager	No
12	Lex	28	Doctor	No
13	Brian	43	Manager	No
14	Ethan	52	Teacher	No
15	Nathan	35	Consultant	No
16	David	32	Machinist	No
17	Nick	41	Sales manager	No
18	Michael	41	Project Manager	No

Profiles and Demographics of Participants

Female Participants

Women ranged from 25 to 43 years (mean 35 years) at the time of interview. The average age at the time of diagnosis was 25–40 years (mean 32 years). This is slightly above the Australian average age of mothers estimated to be 28 years of age (Australian Institute of Health and Welfare, 2007). Twenty-nine women were married, one was single and had no relationship with the partner after pregnancy, two were separated, and one was divorced. Two women temporarily separated from their partners when they were recovering from PND. The categories of highest level of education were high school (n=8), university or business course (n=17), Bachelor's degrees (n=6), and Master's degrees (n=2). Approximately 50% of women (n=16) had returned to work since having their children. One third of women were on antidepressants (n=11) at the time of interview.

Childhood Experiences

Over one-third of women (9/33) experienced sexual abuse, child sexual abuse (n=8) and rape (as an adult) (n=1). One partner disclosed his wife's history of rape in the focus group when it was not disclosed during her interview. As women were not asked specifically about rape this number could also be higher. The number of women who stated they had no history of child sexual abuse could be higher if they preferred not to disclose or dissociated as a result of their experience.

History of child sexual abuse   8
History of rape as an adult   1

Ten women had fond memories of their childhood. Twenty-three women reported unhappy childhoods, which included physical, emotional, and sexual abuse or neglect, parents with mental illness or alcoholic tendencies, death or chronic illness of a parent, controlling fathers, and feeling rejected by their father or mother.

Unhappy memories of their childhood   23
Happy memories of their childhood   10

Relationship with Their Mothers

Thirteen women had positive relationships with their mothers; they described their relationship as great, fantastic, and very close. The remaining women felt either rejected (n=7), or emotionally distant to their mothers (n=10). Three women's mothers had died – one woman found her mother after an overdose when she was a child, and two mothers died of breast cancer.

Positive relationship with mother   13
Feeling rejected by mother   7
Superficial relationship   10
Mothers died   3

Family History of Mental Illness

Twenty-six women reported a family history of depression or PND. Three women thought one of their parents had some form of undiagnosed depression. Four women had no family history of depression or PND.

Family history of depression or PND   26
Undiagnosed depression in parent   3
No family history   4

Almost half of the women (16/ 33) had mothers who were diagnosed with depression (n = 14), or postnatal depression (n = 2). Following their experience with PND, three women were convinced that their mothers had depression, although never diagnosed. For some women both parents were depressed (n = 3) or their father was depressed (n = 7). Women with siblings with depression or PND (n = 9), grandparents with depression (n = 2), cousins (n = 2), or aunt or uncle (n = 2).

Mother with depression or PND   16
Mother with suspected depression   3
Father with diagnosed depression   7
Both parents with diagnosed depression   3
Parents not diagnosed with depression   4

Six women had a family member who committed suicide:

Mothers who committed suicide   1
Siblings who committed suicide   2
Cousin who committed suicide   1
Grandmother who committed suicide   1
Uncle who committed suicide   1

The gender of those who committed suicide was:

Male   4
Female   2

Information About PND in Antenatal Classes

Over half of the women (17/ 33) received no information about PND in antenatal classes. Many women reported only receiving information about PND when they were diagnosed. Only five women received adequate information about PND, but did not think it would happen to them. Women who received minimal information received a pamphlet for PANDA. Seven women could not remember if they received any information about PND.

Happy with information received 5
Minimal information 4
Not sure 7
Received no information 17

Pregnancy Outcome

The number of viable children that women had ranged from one to three children – women with one child (n=9), two children (n=15), three children (n=9). Over one third of women (n=12) experienced pregnancy loss. Ten women experienced miscarriages – women who had one miscarriage (n=7), two miscarriages (n=2), and three miscarriages (n=1). One woman chose to give her baby up for adoption from a previous marriage.

Miscarriages (pregnancy loss to 20 weeks) 10
Foetal death in-utero (FDIU) 1
Stillbirth of an anencephalic baby 1
Baby put up for adoption 1

Women in this study had children that ranged in age from 6 weeks to 14 years. Three partners had children from previous marriages.

Childbirth Experiences

The women delivered a total of sixty-six children, with an average of two each. The numbers below represent the number of births, not women for each type of delivery. Most of the births (46/66) were normal vaginal deliveries, and 20/66 women needed assistance with their deliveries. The number of births that resulted in normal vaginal deliveries were (n=46), emergency caesarean sections (n=9), elective caesareans (n=1), forceps deliveries (n=8), and vacuum extractions (n=2).

Normal vaginal deliveries 46
Emergency caesareans 9
Elective caesareans 1
Forceps deliveries 8
Vacuum extractions 2

Although intervention is not always associated with a traumatic birth experience, women in this category described their births as very painful, shocking, felt like a failure, frightened, out of control, sheer hell, nightmare, horrendous, and a shock.

Women with positive birth experience used terms such as 'pleasurable', 'brilliant', and 'wonderful' when talking about their deliveries.

Traumatic birth experience   21
Positive birth experience   12

Eleven women reported an attachment to their babies. Twenty-two women reported a delay either initially or when they got home from the hospital. Having a baby created feelings of being scared, overwhelmed, disappointed with sex of the baby, numb, shocked, and exhausted. One woman cannot remember seeing and holding her baby after the delivery. Although the average length of time for not bonding was 3–4 months, one woman reported a significant delay with bonding for 13 years.

Women who felt attached to their babies   11
Women who reported a delayed attachment   22

Where Did Women Go When They Developed Symptoms?

Over one-third of women (n = 12) were diagnosed with PND by their maternal and child health nurse. Often the women just happened to be taking their baby in for an assessment rather than specifically going in because of symptoms. Over one-third of women were diagnosed with PND by their GP (n = 8) or other health professionals (n = 4), excluding maternal and child health nurses. The woman's mother, partner or neighbour suggested seeing the GP in three cases. Most women (24/33) attended their GP when symptoms developed.

Maternal and child health nurse   12
GP   8
Self-identified   4
Psychologist   2
Obstetrician   1
Mother/baby unit   1
O'Connell (sleep centre)   1
Social worker   1
Mother suggested GP   1
Partner suggested GP   1
Neighbour suggested GP   1

Women's Perceptions of Diagnosis

Agreed with the diagnosis of PND   18
Ambivalent about the diagnosis   14

Screening

Two-thirds of women (n = 22) were screened for PND by a health professional using the EPDS. In one case one woman had to write answers also. In all cases the EPDS was used. Women who were not screened (n = 9) were diagnosed with PND following an interview. Two women could not remember if a screening tool was used.

EPDS used to diagnose	22
No screening tool used	9
Not sure if screening tool used	2

The Number of Episodes of PND

Twenty-four women had one episode of PND, eight women had two episodes, and one woman had three episodes.

One episode of PND	24
Two episodes of PND	8
Three episodes of PND	1

Onset of PND

Thirty three women had 41 episodes of PND. The number represents the number of episodes of PND, not the number of women. Twenty-two episodes of PND occurred from pregnancy to 4 weeks after delivery. Of these women, eight women developed antenatal depression. Eleven women developed PND 2–5 months after delivery and eight women developed symptoms 6 months or more after the birth. None of the women reported an onset of symptoms 10 months or more after the birth.

In pregnancy	8
Immediately after birth	8
Day 3	2
2 weeks	1
4 weeks	3
2 months	4
3 months	3
4 months	4
5 months	0
6 months	4
7–8 months	3
9 months	1
Over 10 months	0

Duration of PND

Women had difficulty knowing how long PND lasted as it was a gradual process both going into and coming out of depression. When asked 'roughly how long it lasted' women stated the following. Out of 41 experiences of PND, women were able to talk about a definite end in 35 episodes of PND. The number below represents the number of episodes, not the number of women.

Less than 6 months	4
6–12 months	9
18 months	9
2 years	8
3 years	2
4 years	1
6 years	1
8 years	1

Support

Twenty-two women perceived a lack of support from parents, health professionals, family and friends when they recalled their experience of PND. An important finding was that only fifteen women felt supported by their partner when they were experiencing PND.

Women who felt supported by their partners	15
Women who felt they were not supported by their partners	18

Male Participants

The partners of the female participants ranged in age from 26 to 59 years (mean 38 years). The eighteen partners who were involved in this study, their highest education level was high school (n=7), university (n=5), Bachelor's degrees (n=6), and Master's degrees (n=0). Seventeen fathers were working full-time, and one was working part-time (4 days a week).

Men and Depression

Five partners were diagnosed with depression by a health professional. A significant finding was that two partners developed depression when their wife recovered; both of these partners were suicidal, and the other had a history of chronic depression.

Partners with chronic depression   3
Partners who developed depression after PND   2

Appendix C: Resources

Australia
National helplines

AUSTRALIAN BREAST FEEDING
ASSOCIATION 1800 MUM 2 MUM
(1800 686 2 686)

Beyond Blue	1300 22 4636
Domestic Violence	
Lifeline	13 11 14
Mensline	1300 789 978
Panda	1300 726 306
Relationships Australia	1300 364 277

Australian Capital Territory

Domestic Violence	(02) 6280 0900
Parentline	(02) 6287 3833
Queen Elizabeth II Family Centre	(02) 6205 2333
Sexual Assault	(02) 6247 2525

New South Wales

Australian Breast Feeding Association	(02) 8853 4900
Domestic Violence	1800 656 463
Karitane Family Services	1300 227 464
Parentline	13 20 55
Sexual Assault (Sydney)	9819 6565
Sexual Assualt (Rural)	1800 424 017
Tresillian Family Care Centres	1800 637 357
Women's Information and Referral Service	1800 817 227

Northern Territory

Australian Breast Feeding Association	(08) 8411 0301
Domestic Violence	1800 019 116
Parentline	1300 301 300
Sexual Assualt (Darwin)	(08) 8922 7156
Sexual Assault (Alice Springs)	(08) 8951 5880

Queensland

Child Health Line	13 Health
Domestic Violence	1800 811 811
Ellen Barron Early Parenting Centre	1300 366 039
Parentline	1300 301 300
Positive Parenting Program	1300 366 039
Stillbirth And Neonatal Death Support Society (SANDS)	1800 228 655
Sexual Assault	1800 010 120
Women's Infolink	1800 364 277

South Australia

Child, Adolescent and Women's Health Service	1300 364 100
Domestic Violence	1800 800 098
Parent Helpline	1300 364 100
Stillbirth And Neonatal Death Support Society (SANDS)	(08) 8277 0304
Sexual Assault	1800 817 421
Torrens House (Residential)	1300 733 606
Women's Information Service	1800 188 158

Tasmania

Domestic Violence	1800 633 937
Parentline	1800 808 178
Sexual Assault (Southern)	6231 1811
Sexual Assault (Northern)	6334 2740
Sexual Assault (North West)	6431 9711

Victoria

Domestic Violence (Melbourne)	(03) 9373 0123
Domestic Violence (Rural)	1800 015 188
Maternal and Child Health Line (24 h)	13 22 29
Men's Referral Service	1800 065 973
O'Connell (Residential)	(03) 9882 2326
PANDA (Post and Antenatal Depression Assoc)	1300 726 306
Parent Infant Research Institute (PIRI)	(03) 9496 4496

Parentline	13 22 89
Queen Elizabeth (Residential)	(03) 9549 2777
Sexual Assault	1800 806 292
Stillbirth And Neonatal Death Support Society (SANDS)	(03) 9899 0218
Suicide Helpline Victoria	1300 651 251
Tweddle (Residential)	(03) 9689 1577
Women's Information and Referral	1300 134 130

Western Australia

Domestic Violence	1800 007 339
Ngala Family Resource Centre	1800 111 546
Parentline	1800 654 432
Sexual Assault	1800 199 888
Women's Information Service	1800 199 174

United Kingdom

Association for Post Natal Illness	0207 386 0868
Mind Info Line	0845 766 0163
Relate	0845 456 1310
Samaritans	0845 790 9090

Canada

| Motherisk | (416) 813 6780 |

South Africa

Postnatal Depression Support Association (PNDSA)	
National Help Line	+27 (0)82 882 0072
Cape Town	+27 (0)21 797 4498
Gauteng	+27 (0)82 429 2279

United States Of America

| Postpartum Support International | 1 800 944 4773 |
| The MGH Center For Women's Mental Health | (617) 724 7792 |

WEBSITES

Breastfeeding:

http://www.breastfeeding.asn.au
Australian Breastfeeding Association
http://www.llli.org/
La Leche League International – breast feeding support

Infant and child nutrition:

http://www.goforyourlife.vic.gov.au/
A Victorian Government initiative which aims to promote healthy eating and increase
levels of physical activity.
http://www.chw.edu.au
Children's Hospital at Westmead

Maternal health:
http://beyondblue.org.au
Depression/ postnatal depression, Beyond Blue National Postnatal Depression
Initiative
http://www.marcesociety.com/
Marce Society.
http://www.panda.org.au/
Post and Ante Natal Depression Association
http://www.rwh.org.au/wellwomens/
The Women's Hospital, Melbourne

Men's health:
http://www.menslineaus.org.au/
Men's Line Australia
http://www.mrs.org.au/
Men's Referral Service

Parenting:
http://raisingchildren.net.au/
An Australian parenting website for children up to 8 years of age
http://www.cyh.sa.gov.au
Child and Youth Health, South Australia.
http://www.circleofsecurity.org/
An early intervention program for parents and children to assist with attachment
http://goodbeginnings.net.au
Good beginnings parenting support
http://www.anglicarevic.gov.au/parentzone
Parentzone, parenting courses
http://www.positiveparenting.com/
Positive parenting
www.peaceofmindparentingsupport.com.au
Links and resources to help with parenting.
http://www.postpartumprogress.com/about.html

Postpartum Progress offers comprehensive information available on the latest research,
events and resources, as well as personal stories about postpartum depression.

Appendix D: Sue Evans Fund for Families

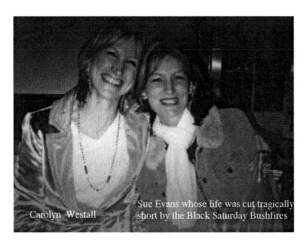

Carolyn Westall (left) with Sue.

Sisters do not come much closer than Sue and Carolyn. Their photo portrays their kinship, friendship and love. They shared their lives and their dreams. Their hearts were sufficiently full as to look to the needs of others. Sue and Carolyn were going to start a charity together before the bushfires. To make their dream a reality, Carolyn has taken the baton alone and is following through on their planned dream – Sue Evans Fund for Families. Sue's charity will assist families who are struggling, disadvantaged, isolated, or need additional support, and is currently funding parents' well-being groups in Melbourne, and will fund future editions of the book, 'Surviving Traumatic Grief' to assist people in their recovery from disasters. With each book sold we give four away. We have given away 2,500 books of the first edition. Future editions will include helping children to cope with traumatic grief.

One-third of the proceeds of this book will go to the Sue Evans Fund for Families. All of the donations into the fund will be used to benefit the community with the aim of reducing depression and postnatal depression.

Carolyn said: 'We would like to be able to help the community in this way, in memory of Sue and her beautiful family'. To donate to this fund or to purchase or find out more about the Surviving Traumatic Grief books please visit the website www.sueevansfund.com.au or send donations to P.O. Box 3126, Eltham, Victoria. 3095. Australia.

Index